FROM
SURVIVING
TO
THRIVING

ISBN PENDING (paperback)
ISBN PENDING (hardcover)
ISBN PENDING (digital)

Lotus Fine Living
lotusellis.com

Printed in the United States of America

FROM
SURVIVING
TO
THRIVING

A Blueprint for Healthy Living

LOTUS ELLIS

Contents

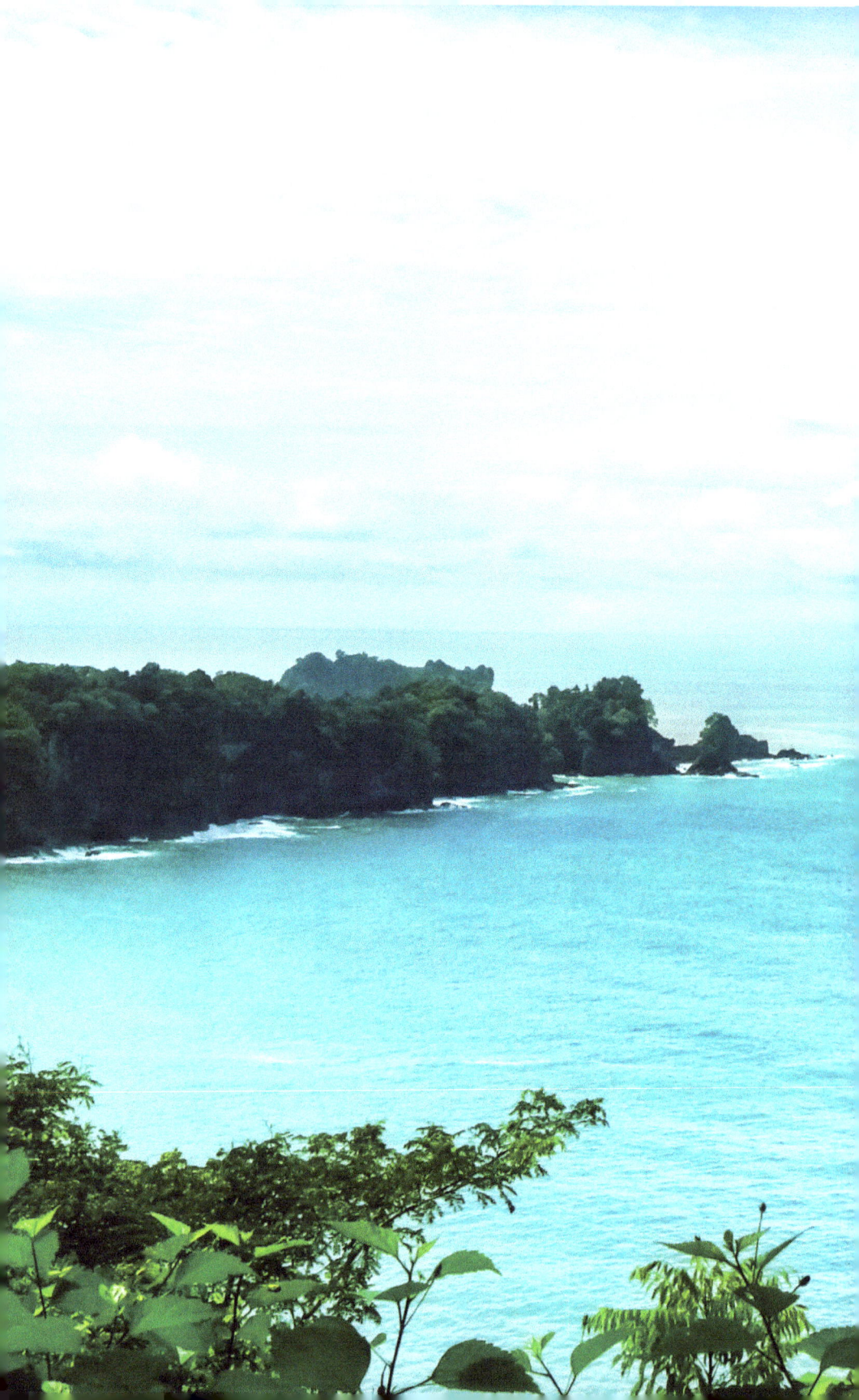

Introduction

'Awareness is the greatest agent of change.'
ECKART TOLLE

In today's modern society, many people don't stop to question whether their food and lifestyle choices are the reason they feel like rubbish. And if some have made that connection, they aren't sure how to make changes that will be impactful and achievable for them.

What you eat, how you manage your stress, and how much you move can reverse certain illnesses and improve overall wellbeing. However, through advertising and social media, everyday brands bombard us with misinformation about what to eat, what to slather on our bodies, and what to clean our homes with. The sad truth is that public health, the health of the planet, and your personal well-being are not at the forefront of marketing. Profit is! I believe that everyone deserves objective, ethically sourced information about how to make choices that protect their health and the environment. And that's what this book is about.

Spending time in Costa Rica, I met an interesting woman named Kelly who had moved down there several years ago to study the country's Blue Zone. Blue Zones are places where people live longer and healthier lives than anywhere else on Earth. The National Institute on Aging has been able to identify these pockets around the world: places where people live to be over 100 and suffer a fraction of the rate of killer diseases that Americans do. Why are people in these places living so long? The secret is lifestyle!

Did you know that twenty-five percent of how long you live is determined by genes and seventy-five percent by lifestyle? Wow! Can that really be? I decided to pick up a copy of *The Blue Zones Solution* by National Geographic researcher Dan Buettner to find out if these centenarians have common traits. The answer is yes! Buettner identified five Blue Zones during more than five years of on-site investigation: the Italian island of Sardinia; Okinawa, Japan; Loma Linda, California; Costa Rica's Nicoya Peninsula; and Ikaria, a Greek island. The people based in these places grow up adhering to a lifestyle that includes a mostly plant-based, healthy diet, daily exercise, low stress, and a sense of purpose.

What do these people eat exactly? Their healthy diet is one that is loaded with vegetables, fruits, fish, and nuts and low in meat, sugar, fat, and the toxic, processed foods of modern civilization. Buettner goes into detail, highlighting several aspects of Blue Zone diets, including local teas and locally grown fruits and vegetables, that seem to be beneficial. The way you eat is important as well as what you eat. At mealtimes, it's recommended you use a smaller vessel since you're likely to eat less if the plate is smaller but fuller. Also, eat more slowly. Eating faster usually results in eating more, which is harder for the body to digest. In the Blue Zones, the biggest meal of the day is typically eaten in the first part of the day or at midday. A smaller meal is taken in the late afternoon or evening. It's also important to focus on the food and be mindful of what you're eating. This is harder if you're watching TV or at your computer.

Your body is a living biological machine. Is it surprising that our bodies suffer when we stuff them with inflammatory, chemically destructive diets high in saturated fat and sugar? The literature shows that a vast volume of cases of heart disease and diabetes can be attributed to a lifetime of obesity and poor diet. It has been documented in thousands of trials and scientific studies that the incidence and severity of several major diseases, including cancer and Alzheimer's, can be severely restricted by a healthy diet.

A daily routine of regular exercise out in nature is another theme that is common across all Blue Zones. The people climb mountains, walk through the hills, work the land, and generally use their bodies in a constant grind as they perform their daily activities. And it doesn't have to be high-intensity exercise either. Often, the exercise is slow and relaxed, but ongoing throughout the day. These people are using their muscles, burning calories, and circulating their blood. Buettner has found that those who live long and healthy in the Blue Zones live low-stress, happy lives enriched with strong family ties, a sense of purpose, spirituality, and plenty of sleep.

To live long and healthy requires a constant, daily lifestyle of positive enrichment for the body and mind. It means finding ways to make healthy food taste good. Finding ways to make exercise a meaningful part of your daily routine. And surrounding yourself with growth-orientated people who share your interest in living a full life that is low in stress, happy, and meaningful.

People are always thinking that complicated medicine and expensive, modern, technological therapies are required to live long and healthy. But a long and healthy life is in the hands of each and every one of us. It is up to each of us to choose a healthy lifestyle.

Create Your Own Vitality Story

After being in the food manufacturing business for over ten years, I decided I needed a reset. I serendipitously found myself in Costa Rica at a yoga instructor retreat — or perhaps I should call it a detox boot camp. This vegan retreat was free of gluten, sugar, and dairy, and booze was prohibited. Yikes! What had I signed up for? Not only was I the oldest person at the retreat, but I was also actually older than most of the participants' parents. I didn't think I would be able to keep up with these twenty-year-old yogis. But, surprisingly, I did! We started our day at 7:00 a.m. with morning journaling, yoga, and meditation. We would enjoy a fresh, organic, detox juice and a vegan breakfast. We studied human anatomy, chakras (the energy channels of the body), yoga sutras, and Ayurveda, and would take part in more yoga practice until about 7:00 p.m. every evening. I felt great! As a matter of fact, I had never felt better. Maybe I was onto something. I decided to stay an extra week, which quickly turned into two.

Maintaining a vegan diet and yogi lifestyle in Costa Rica is very simple. I felt better the longer I spent eating locally grown, fresh produce and being away from modern-day, stressed-out people. I met so many like-minded people who embraced a healthy lifestyle and cared about saving the environment.

One was an incredible woman named Virginia, who had managed to cure herself of Crohn's disease and a very rare blood disorder by changing her diet and mindset. I was very curious how she had managed to pull this off and invited her for tea in hopes of her sharing her story.

She was born in Chile and got on a plane with her family at the age of eight to move to the USA. At the age of twelve, she began to get debilitating pains in her knees, hips, and stomach. She had gone from an active, healthy child to one who was in severe pain. At age fourteen, she fainted, and they ended up taking out her appendix. Come twenty-three years old, she was terminally ill and given little chance of surviving the medical diagnosis of Crohn's disease and Takayasu Arteritis. As a result, she also suffered a stroke and became depressed and bedridden.

Nothing seemed to work, and the doctors told her she would never have children. They recommended removing her colon. In her desperate search, she learned about macrobiotics – an inexpensive method of eating very simply that promised complete regeneration of her digestive system. After a few months on the program, she went from death's door to completely symptom-free. The healing experience brought her knowledge about the workings of her body and the profound connection between digestive illnesses and the food unwell people had been eating. This program also restored her ability to have children (she went on to have two) and gave her back flexibility and a youthful appearance.

Virginia went on to study in order to help others. She consults with clients all over the world. Her focus is showing people that, contrary to what the doctors and current medical education have told them, they can cure their intestinal diseases. Her expertise is in facilitating the healing of the digestive tract at whatever stage or condition it is in. Recognized as one of the leading digestive counselors in the world, she is an author and founder of the Ki of Life Learning Center, a non-profit residential study house launched in 2003. She is active in educating on the prevention of Crohn's and

Colitis. She is a regular speaker at local universities and teaches in Spain, Canada, USA and England. And she has also worked as the head nutritional counsellor at the 5-star Sha Wellness Clinic in Spain, where I've personally had the pleasure of experiencing wonderful treatments, eating delicious meals and taking detox cooking classes.

Taking personal responsibility for what you put in and on your body is the key to rewriting your health story, and this starts with not taking product advertising and marketing at face value. We have all seen numerous examples of well-known brands concealing disturbing health studies about their products from the public. I'm not a conspiracy theorist or a hippie (despite my real name being Lotus and the fact that I did create an organic granola company), but the reality is that the more processed items are, the easier it is to disguise harmful ingredients and the harder digestion becomes.

As an entrepreneur who has studied nutrition, yoga, and meditation practices, I have been a health enthusiast and adventurous home cook for over twenty years. I was inspired to start making cereal at home fifteen years ago because I couldn't find anything that ticked all the nutrition boxes that didn't taste like cardboard. Having started training for triathlons, I was experimenting with an anti-inflammation diet that was free of dairy, gluten, and refined sugar. This identified a gap in the market, and I responded by creating my own organic, vegan, gluten-free cereal company.

Over the years, I've been blessed to receive countless stories from customers and friends who have experienced significant health breakthroughs by eliminating inflammatory foods from their diet and building good gut health to strengthen the immune system. This ignited a passion to create a book that could help everyday people struggling with low energy and health setbacks draw important connections between their diets, mindsets, lifestyle choices, and health symptoms.

My heartfelt intention is to help you feel better, simplify your busy life and get back to basics with simple, healthy recipes and stories that will nourish your mind, body, and soul. These stories and recipes are personal and meaningful to me because they've been gathered from family, friends, and colleagues who also happen to be medical doctors, naturopaths, health pioneers, and mindfulness experts. During the development of this book, I consulted with my cousin Chuck Hughes, the restaurateur and Food Network celebrity chef, to bring you the healthiest and tastiest recipes. I've boiled it all down to create a blueprint that cuts through the misinformation and reduces the overwhelm that comes with making healthy changes to your lifestyle and mindset.

From Surviving to Thriving

My goal is to provide you with easy-access information and resources to help you make better choices. This starts with understanding what all those weird chemical ingredients in your cereal, prepared foods, skin care, and household products are. I'll show you what's toxic and what's not. Where to invest more money on your grocery bill and where you can save money. One of the things that drive me crazy is the fad diets and unhealthy weight-loss products being pushed by influencers and media personalities. I want people to know that it's not a diet that changes things, but a series of gradual changes to their lifestyle. Using my own personal experience and research, I'm including powerful stories and real-life case studies from some amazing people who awakened to their personal truth and created their own vitality story using the blueprint offered in this book.

The book is broken up into two parts:

In Part One: Make Healthier Choices, I guide you to taking back your health by eating right, finding ways to manage stress, and exercising regularly. Great health can be achieved!

In Part Two: Make Healthier Meals, I've mapped it out for you by developing tasty meals you can make at home, with the help of guest contributors like Chuck Hughes and my mother. Preparing healthy meals is easy when you have the tools.

Throughout these pages, I'll show you the important connection between mindset and nutrition. A health crisis can quickly take you down an emotionally dark hole. Illness is like the rock sitting at the bottom of that hole; it looks okay until you pick it up and look underneath to expose all the gunk (poor diet, emotional distress, overwork, lack of self-care, stress, toxic exposure, etc.) By holding it up to the light, you can see the whole picture, and true healing can begin.

One of the things I find most concerning is the increased dependency of people defaulting to prescriptions and surgery to fix a problem before considering dietary changes and functional medicine alternatives. I have personally witnessed many friends and acquaintances transform their health and reverse diagnoses, and believe you have the power to heal by changing your lifestyle.

The essence of my message is that everyone deserves to know the truth... whether it's about the value of avocado oil (good fat is good for you!) or the true impact of too much processed food. You can feel better, live your best life on your terms, and go from surviving to thriving, even if you have troubling health problems like extra weight, ongoing fatigue, allergies, or digestion issues. Let's not forget about the so-called diseases of civilization — cardiovascular disease, cancer, diabetes, autoimmune diseases, and obesity. Maybe you just want to look and feel your best and slow down the onset of aging.

My hope is that these resources, stories, and recipes will inspire and awaken you to a greater possibility for your health and vitality.

I invite you into my home to discover the tools to start your health transformation.

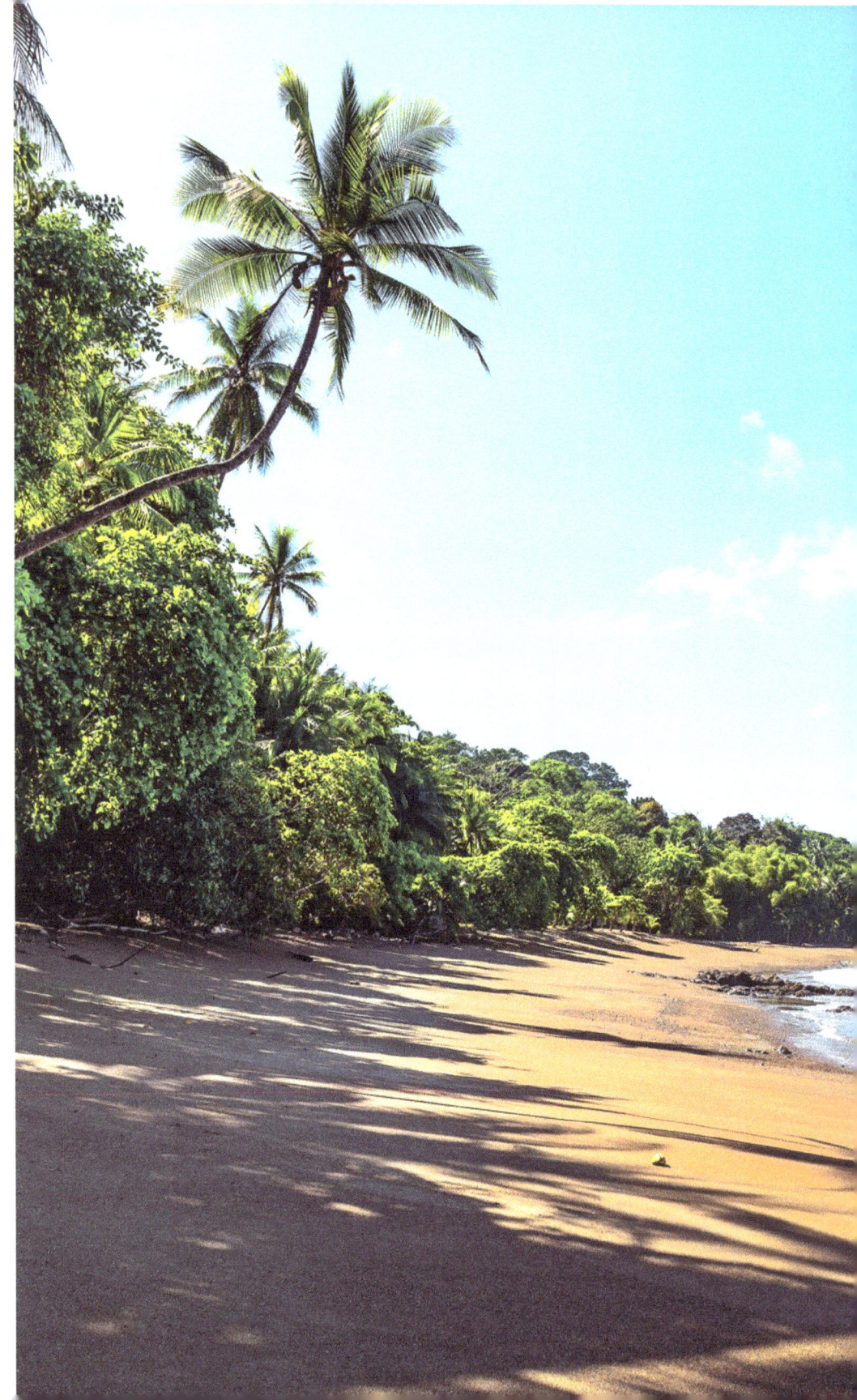

PART ONE

MAKING HEALTHIER CHOICES

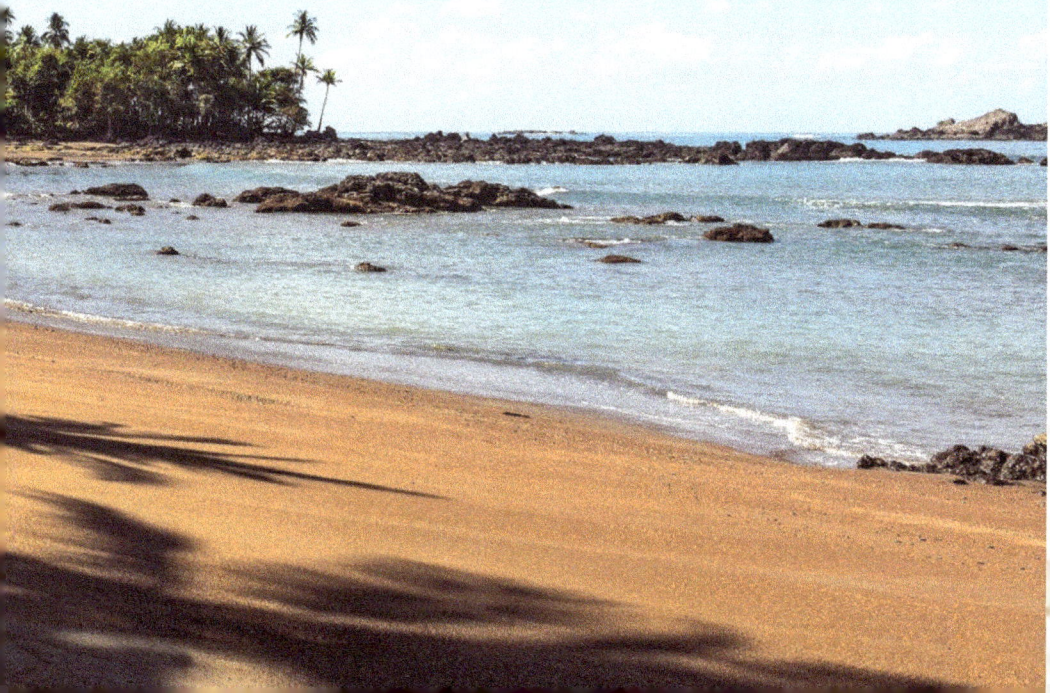

CHAPTER 1

How Does Stress Affect Health?

'All stress comes from resisting what is.'
OPRAH WINFREY

S tress symptoms can affect your body, your thoughts, and your feelings. Being able to recognize common stress symptoms can help you manage them. Ongoing stress can lead to mental health problems and serious medical issues. Stress is associated with high blood pressure, headaches, gastrointestinal problems, anxiety, and depression. It may also worsen skin conditions such as psoriasis and acne, lead to weight gain and make it more difficult to become pregnant.

Stress has many negative psychological and physical health effects; stress management is an important part of maintaining overall health. Eating a healthy diet, regular exercise, meditation, getting out in nature, and finding time for yourself are techniques that help manage stress in your life. Identifying the causes of stress in your life also makes it easier to manage. Once you know your stress triggers, you can identify which triggers can be removed or reduced. You can then focus on coping mechanisms to manage the stressors you cannot change.

Below are some tips for reducing stress in your life. This is some general guidance that you can take away and explore further. The rest of the book focuses on the very first of these tips and goes into detail when it comes to how you can eat well in order to reduce your stress, optimize your health and thrive.

Eat well

Your diet can make a big difference to your mental health. A balanced diet rich in omega-3, organic fruits, vegetables, and whole grains are essential for optimum health, both physical and mental. Good nutrition is an important stress-management tool. Vitamins and minerals work to neutralize harmful molecules produced when your body is under stress and high fiber intake has been associated with greater alertness and decreased perceived stress. The remainder of this book goes into greater detail about how certain foods serve certain purposes and can make you feel good. Feel free to skip ahead to Part Two to try some of the amazing recipes there.

Reduce caffeine, alcohol, and refined sugar consumption

This is a straightforward first step. While many people turn to these for a quick energy boost, caffeine, alcohol and refined sugar are stimulants that increase your stress levels, making it harder to get a restful sleep. Many people use alcohol with the intention of alleviating stress, but it's an unhealthy coping mechanism that just replaces one problem with another. Start by reducing your consumption and aim to replace caffeine drinks with water or herbal teas. Green tea contains healthy antioxidants and less caffeine than coffee.

Get regular physical exercise

The evolutionary 'fight or flight' response is activated when you feel stressed. More adrenalin and cortisol are generated to prepare you for action. Physical exercise metabolizes these excess stress hormones and restores your body to a calm, relaxed state.

Any exercise is better than none at all. Even just taking a walk in nature is a great stress antidote. Try to exercise four to six times a week for half an hour. Including some vigorous exercise like swimming or cycling will get your heart rate up and elevate the benefits.

According to a study published in the Journal of Strength and Conditioning, incorporating strength training can actually lower blood pressure more than aerobic workouts alone. By adding about twenty minutes of weight training to your cardio routine three to five days a week, you'll get blood pressure benefits and build muscle.

Karen's story shows just how much a focus on fitness can change your life.

KAREN'S STORY

I was diagnosed with stage four breast cancer after finding a small tumor near the surface of my breast. After an initial positive prognosis from my doctors, things took a turn for the worse. The cancer had spread, and I faced a survival rate of less than twenty-five percent. I began researching everything I could find and came across information to treat cancer through nutrition. I began a vegan diet and focused on my fitness. I started weightlifting to help maintain my bone mass, running to increase my energy, and yoga to help with my depression.

Cancer destroys your body from the inside out. I had days and weeks where I could barely make it to the bathroom, let alone go for a walk. Running really helped with my energy. when I started, I could barely run for five minutes, but after I got the official remission announcement from my doctor, I ran my first half marathon. I was also dealing with anxiety and depression. Yoga really helped me through those days when I thought I just couldn't go on.

Your health is one of the most important things in your life, and you really need to make time for it. I was too busy with things that ultimately didn't really matter to take care of myself, and I believe that's probably why I wound up with cancer.

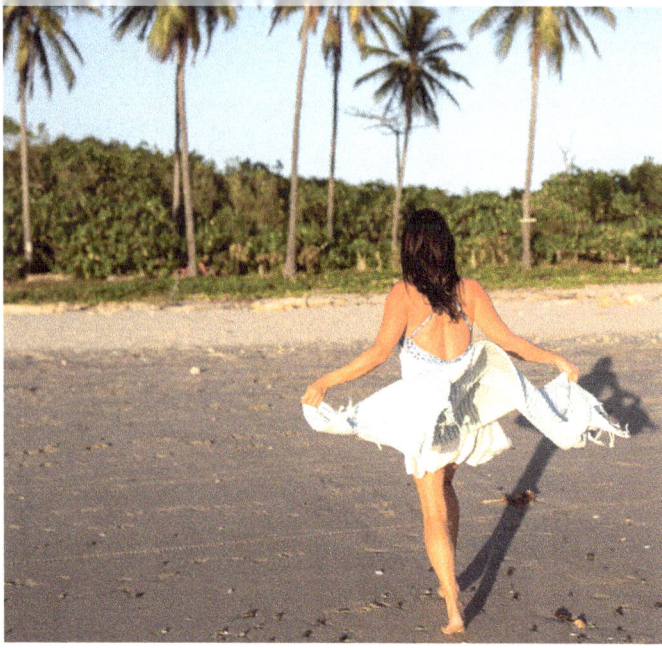

Get out in nature

Spending time in nature can help relieve stress and anxiety, improve your mood and boost feelings of happiness. Humans evolved in the great outdoors, and your brain benefits from a journey back to nature. I love getting out in nature and going for a long hike or getting on my paddle board. The fresh air and exercise help me sleep better too.

Get enough sleep

How much sleep do we really need? According to the National Sleep Foundation (sleepfoundation.org), sleep is a vital indicator of overall health and wellbeing. You need a minimum of seven to eight hours of shut-eye a night. 'Sleep is so incredibly important that no matter how well you eat or how much you exercise, if you are not getting enough rest, the benefits of those healthy lifestyle choices are substantially diminished,' says the co-author Julia Durmer, a sleep medicine and health researcher at Emory University in Atlanta.

Sleep is important for both physical and mental health. Healthy sleep habits can make a big difference in your quality of life. Below are a few helpful tips from the National Sleep Foundation:

14

- Stick to a sleep schedule of the same bedtime and wake-up time, even on the weekends. This helps to regulate your body clock and could help you fall asleep and stay asleep for the night.

- Practice a relaxing bedtime ritual. A relaxing, routine activity right before bedtime away from bright lights and electronic devices helps separate your sleep time from activities that can cause excitement, stress, or anxiety, which can make it more difficult to fall asleep.

- If you have trouble sleeping, avoid naps. Power napping may help you get through the day, but if you find that you can't fall asleep at bedtime, eliminating even short naps may help.

- Exercise daily. Vigorous exercise is best, but even light exercise is better than no activity. It helps increase time spent in deep sleep, which helps boost immune function, support cardiac stress, and control anxiety.

- Evaluate your room. Your bedroom should be cool – between 15 °C and 20 °C (60 °F and 67 °F). Your bedroom should also be free from any noise and light that can disturb your sleep. Check your room for noises or other distractions. This includes a bed partner's sleep disruptions, such as snoring. Consider using blackout curtains, eye shades, ear plugs, 'white noise' machines, humidifiers, fans, and other devices.

- Sleep on a comfortable mattress and pillows. Make sure your mattress is comfortable and supportive. The one you have been using for years may have exceeded its life expectancy – about nine or ten years for most good-quality mattresses.

    Have comfortable pillows free of allergens that might affect you.

Talk it out

When you're feeling overwhelmed with stress, it can help to talk to someone. Talking to a close friend or family member can help you gain a new perspective. The mind has a way of playing tricks on us sometimes. Just being aware of what's going on in your mind will help you make better decisions; it will help you step back from emotionally charged, difficult situations so that you can respond rather than react. If you talk about it, you can change your perception. If you still feel overwhelmed with the stress, your healthcare provider may be able to suggest a mental health professional you can speak to.

Practice yoga

As a certified yoga instructor, I can attest that yoga provides instant gratification and lasting transformation. In the fitness world, both are extremely important. Yoga can change your physical and mental capacity quickly while preparing the mind and body for long-term health. Most yoga studios and local gyms offer yoga classes that are open to all generations and fitness levels. Yoga is for all ages, whether you are ninety, forty, or even thirteen, yoga can help you too. Try going to yogajournal.com and explore yoga 101.

Yoga encourages overall health and wellness and is not just about working out; it's about a healthy lifestyle. The practice of yoga allows students to find stillness in a world consumed with chaos. Peace and tranquility are achieved through focused training. Yoga's deep breathing and meditation practices help relieve stress and declutter the mind, helping you to become more focused.

Yoga's focus on strength and flexibility is of incredible benefit to your body. The postures are meant to strengthen your body from the inside out, so you don't just look good; you feel good, too. Each of the yoga poses is built to reinforce the muscles around the spine, the very center of your body, which is the core from which everything else operates. When the core is working properly, posture is improved, helping to alleviate back, shoulder, and neck problems.

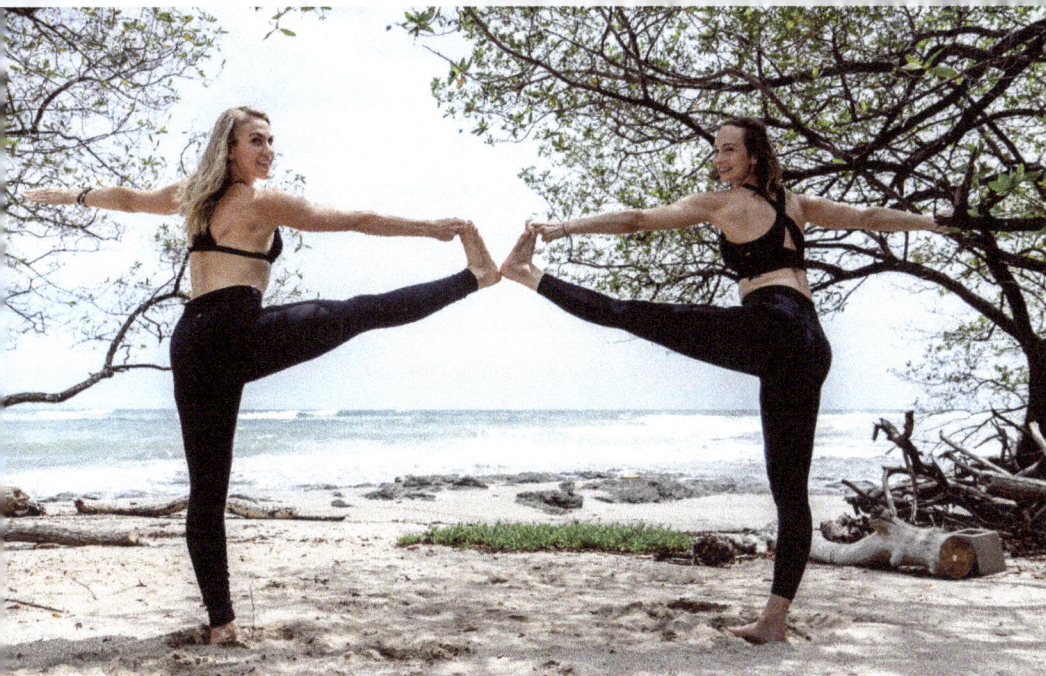

Mary's story shows how practicing yoga and meditation can lead to having a better relationship with your body.

MARY'S STORY

I was first introduced to yoga in the hospital. I had attempted suicide multiple times and was ill with anorexia. I was in a terrible state and had lost over half my body weight. This was a year ago now, and today I am infinitely better. A big part of my recovery is down to yoga.

At first, I didn't take it seriously at all, but actually, I found that it kind of empowered me to realize my body isn't just what people can see, but how I can use it.

My first yoga session was a turning point. It was a very slow class because it was at a treatment facility. I couldn't move beyond a few stretches. I didn't realize how physical and complex it could be. It was introduced to me as a way to calm. Yoga also helped to introduce me to meditation.

I have always been flexible because I used to be a gymnast and dancer. Maybe that's why I developed an eating disorder. But yoga and meditation made me realize that it's not just about my appearance, but also what I can do with my body. I can do headstands and can now meditate for an hour. When I first started, I could barely sit and meditate for ten minutes.

Life is now so much better. My mental health has vastly improved. I am able to maintain friendships and will be going back to school in September. I was an over-thinker and analyzed everything, which made me very anxious most of the time. The clarity of yoga was really what helped make that mind-body connection. It has really helped me stay grounded and being more in the present has taught me how to stay calm.

Practice meditation and breathing (Pranayama in yogic tradition)

With the hectic pace and demands of modern life, many people feel stressed and overworked. Our stress and tiredness make us unhappy, impatient, and frustrated. We are often so busy we feel there is no time to stop and meditate. But meditation actually gives you more time by making your mind calmer and more focused. A simple ten- or fifteen-minute breathing meditation, as explained below, can help you to overcome your stress and find some inner peace and balance.

Meditation can also help us to understand our own minds. We can learn how to transform our minds from negative to positive and from unhappy to happy. Overcoming negative thoughts and cultivating positive thoughts is the purpose of the transforming meditations found in the Buddhist tradition. This profound spiritual practice can be practiced throughout the day, not just while seated. We feel relaxed when we take slower and deeper breaths. Taking a

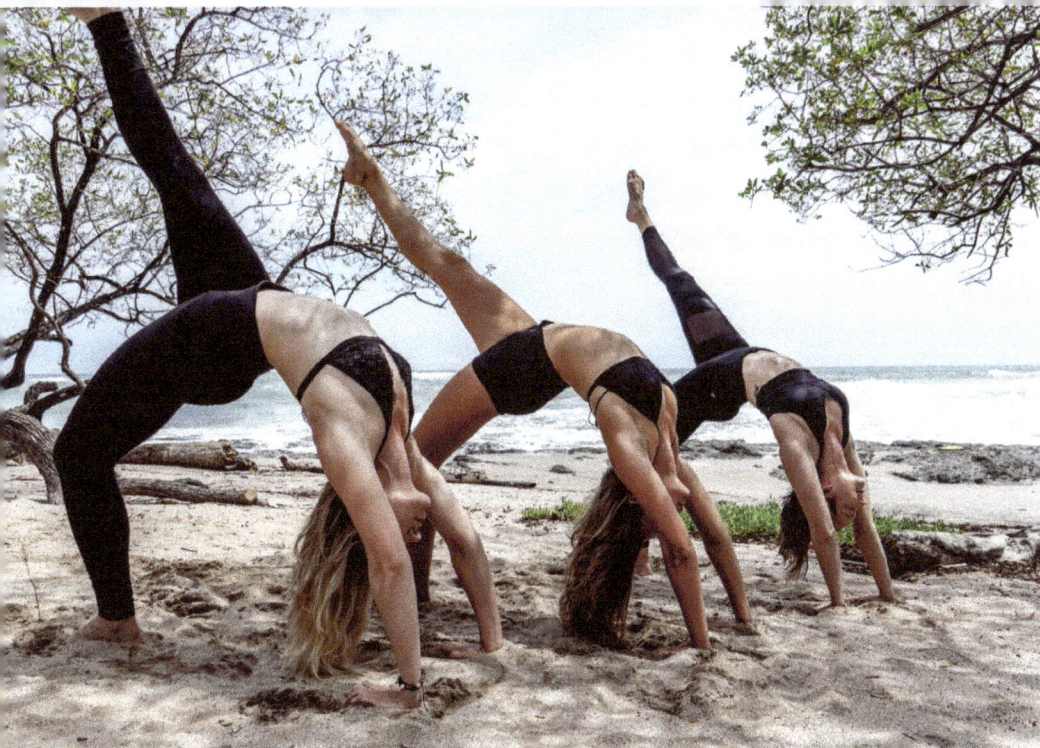

moment to focus on your breath and practice deep breathing can help your mind and body feel calm and relaxed. Taking time out of your busy day to meditate and calm down can be extremely beneficial for managing stress and anxiety.

If you can slow down your mind and body long enough to realize that you are not in mortal danger, you will remain calm. One way to do this is by breathing deeply or using a mantra technique – a repeated slogan or phrase. Relaxation lowers your pulse rate, respiration, and blood pressure. When you combine different techniques such as deep breathing, muscle relaxation, meditation, and yoga, you can significantly lower your stress levels. You will also elevate your mood and improve your ability to focus.

Try the following breathing exercises:

Belly breath

With one hand on your belly, relax your abdominal muscles and slowly inhale through the nose, bringing air into the bottom of your lungs. You should feel your abdomen rise. Continue to inhale as your rib cage expands outward. At the peak of the inhalation, pause for a moment, then exhale gently from the top of your lungs to the bottom. At the end of the exhalation, contract your abdominal muscles slightly to push residual air out of the bottom of your lungs.

Ocean's breath

Also known as Ujjayi, this will immediately soothe and settle your mind. Take an inhalation that is slightly deeper than normal. With your mouth closed, exhale through your nose while constricting your throat muscles. If you are doing this correctly, you should hear a sound like waves on the ocean and feel the outflow of air through your nasal passages.

Alternate nostril breathing

Known as balancing breath, or Nadi Shodhana in the yogic tradition, this will immediately help you feel calmer. Hold your right thumb over your right nostril and inhale deeply through your left nostril. At the peak of your inhalation, close off your left nostril with your fourth finger, lift your right thumb, and then exhale smoothly through your right nostril. After a full exhalation, inhale through the right nostril. At the peak of your inhalation, close off your right nostril with your thumb, lift your fourth finger and exhale smoothly through your left nostril. Continue for five minutes.

Practice Qi Gong

What is Qi Gong? It can be described as a mind-body-spirit practice that improves one's mental and physical health by integrating posture, movement, breathing technique, self-massage, sound, and focused intent. Qi Gong opens the flow of energy in meridians used in acupuncture and Chinese medicine. It enhances our ability to feel the Life Force underlying the physical world and to deepen our communication with it. Physically slow, gentle Qi Gong movements warm tendons, ligaments, muscles, vital organs, and connective tissue. The National Qigong Association (www.nqa.org) is a wonderful resource helping individuals find a path to support their goals and to evolve this amazing, energetic science.

Find what works for you!

There are many techniques for managing stress and different things work for each person. Incorporating one or more of these techniques into your daily routine can greatly reduce your stress levels and improve your quality of life. Just adding as little as ten minutes of daily meditation, taking a five-minute break to focus on your breath, and dedicating thirty minutes to exercise daily can have a dramatic effect on reducing stress.

CHAPTER 2

Nourishing the Body

'America is eating too many processed foods
loaded with chemicals, simple carbohydrates,
and fats designed in laboratories.'

ALEGANDRO JUNGER, MD

About eighty percent of what you find on supermarket shelves today didn't exist 100 years ago. At a time when people are very concerned with their health and its relationship to what they eat, we have handed over the responsibility for our nourishment to faceless corporations. By creating healthy meals each day using fresh ingredients from clean food sources, you reclaim control over your health.

There is a lot of confusion out there about which foods and products are healthy, and which are not. One of the most important things you can do to be healthier is to read labels. This applies to all foods, even so-called health foods. Choose real whole foods which are low in sugar and high in fiber. Buy organic and local foods which are free from hormones and antibiotics whenever possible. Choose grass-fed meat and wild sustainable fish if you eat meat.

Why is this so important? Our bodies are so overloaded with toxins in our daily lives—from the water we drink and shower in, to the products we use on our skin, to the food we eat. The best way to reduce your exposure is to eat safer food and use the healthiest beauty products whenever possible. It is a known fact that toxins take the biggest toll on growing children, whose developing bodies are far more affected by the amounts they consume on an everyday basis.

Investing in a good water filtration system

Tap water today can carry many toxins. It is often treated with fluoride to strengthen teeth, which can be linked to problems with kidneys, thyroid, and central nervous system. It is treated with chlorine to kill microscopic organisms. And it can contain lead. In fact, it's so toxic that almost all of your body organs will be affected by it.

Meanwhile, arsenic naturally occurring in certain types of rocks can contaminate groundwater and underground reservoirs. This kind of arsenic poisoning is common in many parts of the world. A major source of the arsenic in water is mining and industrial pollution. Golf courses and large-scale agriculture also use heavy fertilizers and pesticides, which leach into the groundwater. And many drugs used in the medical field are finding their way into our groundwater systems, eventually ending up in our tap water. These include over-the-counter drugs commonly used for pain relief as well as prescription drugs. Patients taking the drugs usually excrete large amounts of them in urine. They reach groundwater from the sewage.

Water filtration systems come in many different shapes and prices. It's important to select a water filtration system that suits your water condition. To do that, you need to know the problem. It's best to have your water tested to give you a starting point. The pH (measurement of acidity or alkalinity in a substance) of pure water is seven. In general, water with a pH lower than seven is acidic, and water with a pH greater than seven is considered alkaline. The pH range for groundwater and foods should be around seven and above.

There is more to water filtration than just purity. The right type of filter can promote better health. Options, depending on your needs, include a reverse osmosis under-sink filter, a volcanic rock mineral filtration system, an alkaline countertop water filter, or a simple water filtration pitcher.

Why buy organic?

I recently attended a talk given by the Rodale Institute Chief Impact Officer explaining that choosing to buy organic isn't just about food.

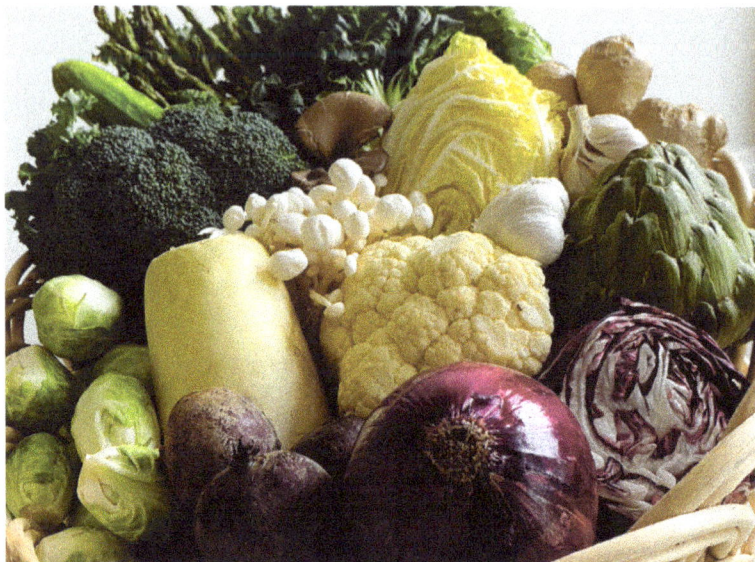

We were told, 'Conventional and organic farming methods have different consequences on the environment and people. Conventional agriculture causes increased greenhouse gas emissions, soil erosion, water pollution, and threatens human health. Organic farming has a smaller carbon footprint, conserves and builds soil health, replenishes natural ecosystems for cleaner water and air, all without toxic pesticide residues.'

But are organic foods worth the extra money? In most cases, yes. Buying organic when it comes to certain items may lower your exposure to chemicals. In other cases, it may not be worth the money. Some basic information can help you make smarter choices.

I love talking to people about food. And these days, I inevitably end up talking about GMOs. Genetically modified crops, worldwide, have been engineered to tolerate being sprayed with glyphosate herbicides. Glyphosate tolerance is a trait that allows farmers to spray the GM crops and kill the weeds but not the corn or soy, peanuts, and oats. Choosing organically grown crops allows you to avoid exposure.

A new report issued by the President's Cancer Panel recommends eating produce without pesticides to reduce your risk of getting cancer and other diseases. According to the Environmental Working Group (an organization of scientists, researchers, and policymakers), certain types of organic produce can reduce the amount of toxins you consume on a daily basis by as much as eighty percent.

'The Dirty Dozen' and 'The Clean 15' are lists that help consumers know when they seriously should buy organic. These lists were compiled by the United States Government's Pesticides Data Program Reporting, a pesticide residue monitoring system enacted back in 1991. Every year, a new report is released.

The Dirty Dozen 2021

The fruits and vegetables on the 'Dirty Dozen' list, when conventionally grown, tested positive for at least forty-seven different chemicals, with some testing positive for as many as sixty-seven. Because these crops have the highest levels of contamination, the Environmental Working Group suggests you buy these twelve crops organic when possible.

1. Strawberries
2. Spinach
3. Kale and Collard Greens
4. Nectarines
5. Apples
6. Grapes
7. Cherries
8. Peaches
9. Pears
10. Peppers
11. Celery
12. Tomatoes

The Clean 15 2021

All the produce on 'The Clean 15' list bore little to no traces of pesticides and are safe to consume in non-organic form.

1. Avocados
2. Sweet corn
3. Pineapples
4. Onions
5. Papayas
6. Sweet peas (frozen)
7. Eggplant
8. Asparagus
9. Broccoli
10. Cabbage
11. Kiwifruit
12. Cauliflower
13. Mushrooms
14. Honeydew melons
15. Cantaloupe

Why are some types of produce more prone to sucking up pesticides than others? As Richard Wiles, Senior Vice President of Policy for the Environmental Working Group, comments, 'If you eat something like a pineapple, it has a protection defence because of the outer layer of skin. Not the same for strawberries and berries.'

The President's Cancer Panel recommends washing conventionally grown produce to remove residues. Wiles adds, 'You should do what you can do . . . the idea you are going to wash pesticides off is a fantasy. But you should still wash it because you will reduce pesticide exposure.'

There is a full list containing forty-nine types of produce, rated on a scale of least to most pesticide. You can check out the full list on the Environmental Working Group's website at www.foodnews.org.

Making healthier food choices and promoting good gut bacteria

By far the simplest way to eat healthily and lose weight is to avoid refined sugar and processed foods. Read the nutritional tables to really understand what you're eating and pay attention to portion control. A good rule to remember is that real food doesn't need an ingredient list, because real food is the ingredient. The rise in chronic diseases linked to obesity is one of the most important public health issues facing our society today, from diabetes and heart disease to certain kinds of cancers and breathing disorders. Obesity is on the rise, so understanding the underlying metabolic causes of weight gain, and how to correctly measure energy intake and expenditure, is extremely important. We need to regulate our own consumption patterns while avoiding the many weight-loss gimmicks that exist today. When it comes to ongoing health and wellbeing, Nicky's story demonstrates just how radical a change can be caused by focusing on what you do and don't put in your body.

NICKY'S STORY

I was diagnosed with type 1 diabetes as a child. I was taught about medication, not nutrition. I believed that as long as I took my insulin, I could eat and drink whatever I wanted. I was so wrong!

At age forty, I was diagnosed with hypothyroidism and hypertension. At fifty, I was diagnosed with rheumatoid arthritis and osteoarthritis. I was given cortisone shots, which raised my blood sugar astronomically and caused me to gain weight. I reached 90 kilos (199 pounds)! I was spinning out of control and something needed to change ASAP.

I became determined to get better. I gave up eating all animal products, refined sugar, processed foods, and refined carbohydrates. I ate vegetables, whole grains, beans, nuts, and all seeds I could find.

Within three months, I lost thirty pounds. My cholesterol stabilized, so my doctor took me off of my cholesterol medication. Within six months, I had dropped another twenty pounds, and he took me off the blood pressure pills and my insulin prescription was cut in half. My joint pain lessened. A whole-food, plant-based diet turned my life around. I've never felt or looked younger. I enjoy sharing my journey and letting others know that it's not hard to make the change; all we need to do is make better choices.

So, if you want to follow Nicky's example and make healthier choices, what foods should you avoid or at least minimize?

Sugar

Added sugar is the single worst ingredient in the modern diet. However, some sources of sugar are worse than others. Refined sugars are well known for giving your body a temporary boost and then causing an energy crash which leaves you feeling tired and irritable. When consumed in large amounts, sugar can drive insulin resistance in the body and is strongly linked to non-alcoholic fatty liver disease. It is also associated with various serious diseases, including type 2 diabetes and heart disease.

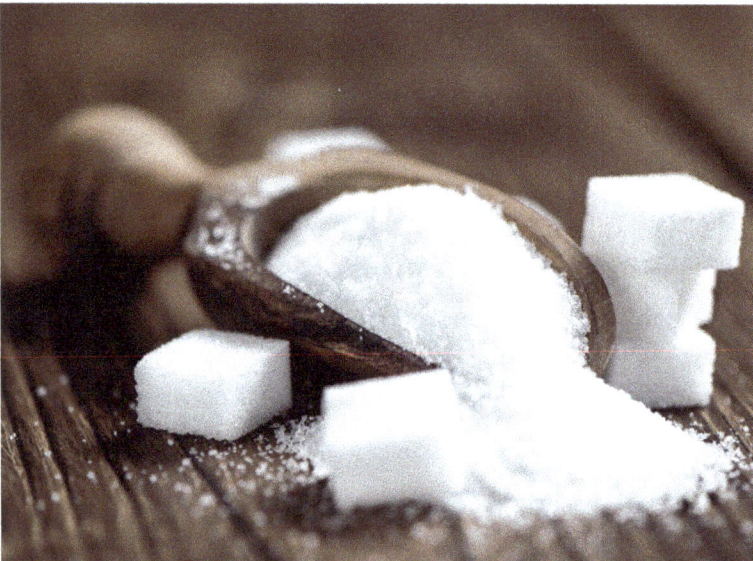

When it comes to adding sugar to your food and drink, there are alternatives: Stevia is natural, calorie-free, and does not affect blood sugar. This is an option for people who are concerned with blood sugar or calories. Maple syrup and honey are a better alternative to white sugar or corn syrup (as it contains trace minerals). However, it is not suggested that you consume these products daily.

Fruit juice is often assumed to be healthy, but this is a mistake. Many fruit juices are actually little more than fruit-flavored sugar water. It is true that the juice contains some antioxidants and vitamin C, but this must be weighed against a large amount of liquid sugar. Sugary carbonated beverages contain phosphoric acid, which contributes to many serious health dangers that include lowering bone density, tooth decay, major kidney issues, decrease of nutrients in the body, and increased body acidity.

There are some fruit juices that have been shown to have health benefits despite the sugar content, such as pomegranate juice and blueberry juice. However, mixing a little water or tea with the juice can be a great solution to cut the sugar while keeping the antioxidants.

Refined carbohydrates

We've been taught to stay far away from them, but not all carbohydrates are bad. Refined carbohydrates, which have a higher glycemic index than unprocessed carbs, are the ones that cause inflammation in our bodies. Refined carbohydrates have been stripped of their fiber. Fiber promotes fullness, improves blood sugar control, and feeds the beneficial bacteria in your gut. Good carbs are plant foods, whole grains, beans, fruits, and vegetables. Bad carbs are refined 'white' grains like white bread and rice.

White bread and pastries are generally made with refined sugar, refined wheat flour, and added fats, which are often disturbingly unhealthy fats like shortening and margarine (high in trans fats). These foods are some of the worst things that you can put into your body; they have almost no nutrients but tons of calories, and contain the protein gluten. For this reason, all wheat-based products are a bad idea for people with gluten sensitivity. They can be debilitating for those with celiac disease. The majority of them are made from refined wheat, which is low in essential nutrients (while high in empty calories) and leads to rapid spikes in blood sugar.

Most conventional wheat is also sprayed with glyphosate, which is an herbicide that is used to control grass weeds prior to planting and after wheat is harvested. Glyphosate has come under increased scrutiny in the past year. The World Health Organization's cancer group, the International Agency for Research on Cancer, classifies the herbicide as a probable carcinogen. There is growing research that glyphosate is an endocrine disruptor and also kills beneficial bacteria which your gut needs.

When it comes to the alternatives, for people who can tolerate gluten, Ezekiel bread is an excellent choice. Whole grain or sprouted grain is also definitely better (or less bad for you) than white bread.

Bad oils

Decrease consumption of refined vegetable oils, such as soybean oil, corn oil, and cottonseed oil. These oils are very high in omega-6 fatty acids, which humans have never consumed in such large amounts before. There are many serious concerns with these oils. They are highly sensitive to oxidation and cause increased oxidative stress in the body. They have also been linked to an increased risk of cancer. All poly and monounsaturated fats (oils that are liquid at room temperature) oxidize when exposed to heat, light, and oxygen. The oils listed above are produced using high heat, which means they have been oxidized and are carcinogenic. This is a major reason to choose oils that are cold-pressed rather than extracted by using heat.

Healthier oils

Nut and seed oils – These are flavorful and a great ingredient to add to your recipes. Oils derived from nuts are very healthy. Coldpressed flaxseed and walnut oil are rich in alpha-linolenic acid (ALA), a plant-based omega-3 fatty acid your body can't make. Both plant- and fish-based omega-3s are great for lowering elevated triglyceride levels, lowering your risk of heart disease, joint pain, depression, and brain health. Flaxseed oil should be consumed at room temperature, so in salad dressings and smoothies. Sesame

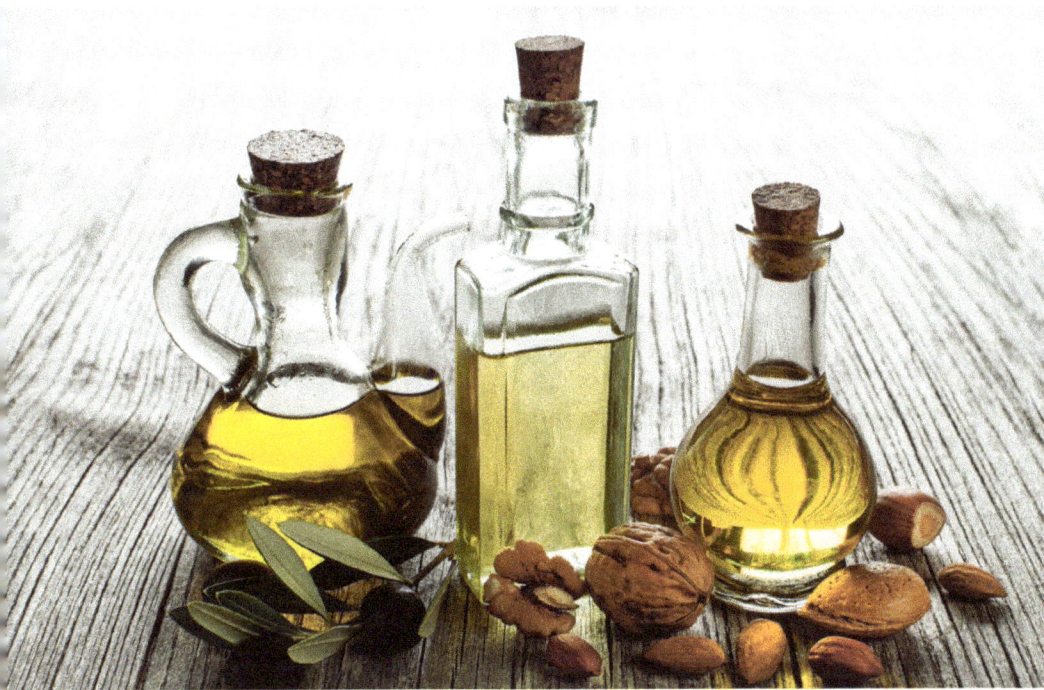

oil is another delicious option, with strong anti-inflammatory properties. It's my favorite for Asian-inspired recipes.

Avocado oil — This has a particularly high smoke point (270 °C or 520 °F), making it a great option when cooking at high temperatures. Avocados are loaded with many nutrients, many of which are lacking in the modern diet. They are weight-loss-friendly and heart-healthy. According to a study published in The Journal of Nutrition, adding avocado oil to your salsa can help you absorb the antioxidants. The researchers saw a similar bump in nutrient absorption when they added avocado oil to a salad, too. That's because carotenoids are fat-soluble, meaning your body actually needs the help of fat to fully absorb them. Fat-soluble vitamins A, D, E, and K also require fat to be digested.

Extra virgin olive oil — This oil is a universal favorite for a reason. It's a staple of the heart-healthy Mediterranean diet, which research shows may benefit your brain, eyes, kidneys, and skin. The monounsaturated fats in olive oil have also been shown to reduce your low-density lipoprotein (LDL) cholesterol, or bad cholesterol. The smoke point is pretty low, so it tends to burn easily. This can damage the good-for-you fat in the oil and mess with the flavor, so stick to low or medium heat.

Processed meat and corn-fed red meat

Fatty red meats are considered inflammatory perpetrators which have been linked to various health conditions, such as chronic diabetes, heart disease, and cancer, according to several medical studies, including those most recently out of the University of California, San Francisco. Corn and soy-fed cows develop gastric inflammation and infections, and they need antibiotics. When we eat their meat, we are eating the inflammation, which makes us more prone to coronary artery disease, cancer, and other chronic diseases.

Processed deli meats can contain a wide variety of additives, from nitrates to carrageenan, which can increase inflammation in the body and have been scientifically linked to increased risk of many serious diseases, including cancer, type 2 diabetes, and heart disease.

As an alternative, choose grass-fed beef or eliminate beef and processed meat from your diet altogether.

Milk

It's no surprise that so many people suffer from cow milk intolerance or milk allergy, which is an allergy to casein (milk protein) or lactose (sugar in milk). Cow's milk and cream cheese have been deemed highly inflammatory foods for the amount of stomach upset, constipation, diarrhea, hives, and breathing issues they cause.

If you suffer from a milk intolerance or allergy, there are a number of milk alternatives available. Try swapping animal milk for nut milk. These milk alternatives blend nicely with coffee and in baking, smoothies, and cereal.

Low-fat yogurt

Yogurt can be incredibly healthy. Unfortunately, most yogurts found in the grocery store are extremely bad for you. They are frequently low in fat but loaded with sugar to make up for the lack of taste that the fats provided. The yogurt has had the healthy, natural dairy fats removed, only to be replaced with something much worse. Additionally, many yogurts don't actually contain probiotic bacteria, as generally believed. They have often been pasteurized after fermentation, which kills all the bacteria.

As an alternative, choose plain, full-fat yogurt that contains live or active cultures (probiotics). Choose organic yogurt or try a nut-based vegan yogurt.

Processed cheese

Processed cheese products are not real cheese. They are mostly made with filler ingredients that are combined and engineered to have a similar look and texture to cheese. Read labels, and make sure that the cheese you're eating is actually cheese.

As an alternative, eat organic cheese when possible. Flavorful cheese seems to cause fewer issues. Goat and sheep cheese are a great option as they are easier to digest. Dairy is mucous-forming, so those that suffer from skin issues or lung issues may find that cutting dairy out altogether will resolve these problems.

Fried food

While tasty, french fries and potato chips are very high in calories and easy to eat in excessive amounts. Several studies link the consumption of french fries and potato chips with weight gain. These foods may also contain large amounts of acrylamides, carcinogenic substances that form in foods cooked at high temperatures. The amino acid asparagine in the food reacts with sugars to produce acrylamide. This chemical can form in many fried foods, but it's especially common in potatoes, which are high in sugars like fructose and glucose. Acrylamide has been shown in animal studies to cause cancer. Several studies have linked fried foods to serious health problems like type 2 diabetes and heart disease, due to increased risk factors such as obesity, high blood pressure, and high cholesterol.

Fried foods served in fast-food restaurants are often cooked in hydrogenated oils, which raise bad (LDL) cholesterol levels, lower good (HDL) cholesterol levels, and raise your chance of having heart disease. Hydrogenated oil is especially unhealthy when it's reused, which restaurants often do. Oils break down with each frying, which changes their composition and causes more oil to be absorbed into the food.

Try instead making oven-baked fries using a plain white or sweet potato. You can also pan-fry food with a little olive or avocado oil.

Alcohol (also known as ethanol)

While drinking a glass of red wine a day has health benefits, heavy drinking over time appears to increase the risk of developing chronic diseases and other serious problems, including:

- High blood pressure, heart disease, stroke, liver disease, type 2 diabetes, and digestive problems
- Cancer of the breast, mouth, throat, esophagus, liver, and colon
- Learning and memory problems
- Mental health problems, including depression and anxiety
- Weight gain

So how come a glass of red wine can be good for you? Research suggests it provides antioxidants, helps protect against heart disease, and may promote longevity.

If you do drink wine, choose wines that are low in sugar content. When choosing mixed drinks, go with something that has less sugar, like vodka and club soda, or tequila.

Food additives

We've long heard the warnings about consuming a diet rich in processed foods. These foods have been altered, in some way, from their natural state. Consuming a small amount of some processed foods might be safe, but the health risks add up. One reason is that they contain popular additives, such as monosodium glutamate (MSG), a flavor enhancer commonly added to Chinese foods, canned soups, and processed meats. The FDA has received many reports of adverse reactions to foods containing MSG. These reactions include headaches, numbness or tingling, sweating, heart palpitation, and nausea.

Other additives to think twice about include sodium nitrites, sulfites, trans fats, and yellow dye #5 and #7, which can be found in cereals and candy.

Putting it into practice

This may seem like a lot of information, but the guidance is really simple to put into practice! In summary, fill up on fresh food and minimize processed foods that contain food additives, sugar, and unhealthy oil. Shop at your local farmers' market. Choose frozen fruits and vegetables without additives if fresh foods are not available to you. Read the labels! Check the list of ingredients before adding foods to your grocery cart. Beware of any ingredients you can't pronounce. And then, be your own chef and cook your own meals so you know what you're eating (this is where Part Two comes in!).

CHAPTER 3

Boosting Your Immune System

'All disease begins in the gut.'

HIPPOCRATES, THE FATHER OF MODERN MEDICINE

Your first, and most important, line of defense against getting sick is your lifestyle. Not smoking or drinking heavily, and making sure you are exercising, getting enough sleep, and choosing healthy foods will give you the best shot at a healthy immune system, so you can reduce your chances of getting sick and minimize the severity of an illness if you do.

The immune system is the group of cells and molecules that protect us from disease by monitoring our body and responding to any foreign substances they perceive as threats, particularly infectious microbes. Our immune system works with diverse gut flora, not only to create defenses against pathogens but also to develop a tolerance for beneficial microbes. The immune system and the gut microbiota have developed a mutualistic relationship, regulating one another and cooperating to support each other. The importance of this interaction is highlighted by the fact that seventy to eighty percent of the body's immune cells are found in the gut.

The gut bacteria are known to play a crucial role in keeping us healthy. Research has shown that the trillions of friendly microorganisms hosted by our guts are there to help us. Various studies have been slowly unraveling the complex relationship between gut bacteria and immunity. They suggest that a healthy gut contributes to a strong immune system, heart health, clean skin, brain health, improved mood, healthy sleep, and effective digestion, and it may help prevent some cancers and autoimmune diseases.

The human digestive system, or microbiome, which is home to microscopic cells of bacteria, is made up of good and bad bacteria. The GOOD strains of bacteria, which keep you healthy, metabolize food efficiently to turn nutrients into things your body can use.

Probiotics are part of the good gut microbiome; these boost gastrointestinal health and can make your immune system stronger. You can find them in products like yogurt and kefir. Look for cultures of bacteria like bifidobacteria and lactobacilli when reading labels. They're also found in kombucha and fermented vegetables like kimchi, sauerkraut, and pickled vegetables.

The BAD bacteria strains make you sick, fat, and tired. Studies have found if you have too much of a certain kind of bad bacteria in your gut microbiome, you may suffer from autoimmune disorders and you're more likely to have Crohn's disease, ulcerative colitis, and irritable bowel syndrome (IBS).

Polyphenols found in dark blue and purple plants, red wine, dark chocolate, artichokes, cloves, star anise, cinnamon, cumin, dried peppermint, berries, broccoli, pomegranates, leafy greens, olives, hazelnuts, pecans, chicory, and more are proven to fuel your good gut bacteria. Polyphenols also improve blood vessel function and balance cholesterol levels. Certain vegetables are rich in prebiotic fiber which helps digestion, including chicory root, Jerusalem artichoke, onions, garlic, leeks, rutabagas, asparagus, parsnips, and so on. Gut health influences skin vitality, energy levels, metabolism, moods, brain function, and the ability to fight off disease. Prebiotics are good for probiotics. When you combine the two, it's a symbiotic relationship. The idea behind this is that prebiotics helps the probiotics live longer. You can make symbiotic combinations by having a banana with your morning yogurt.

For the immune system to function well, it requires balance and harmony. There is still much that researchers don't know about the intricacies and interconnectedness of the immune response. Researchers are exploring the effects of diet, exercise, age, psychological stress, and other factors. General healthy-living strategies are a good way to start giving your immune system a boost.

Healthy ways to strengthen your immune system

Following general good-health guidelines is the single best step you can take toward naturally keeping your immune system strong and healthy. You'll notice the crossover with the tips from Chapter One on reducing stress — what is good for one aspect of health is often good for other aspects, so putting these things into practice will have multiple benefits. Every part of your body, including your immune system, functions better when protected from environmental assaults and bolstered by healthy-living strategies such as these:

- Practicing correct handwashing and oral hygiene
- Staying hydrated (drinking eight glasses of water a day)
- Avoiding smoking
- Eating a healthy variety of fruits and veggies
- Maintaining a healthy weight
- Exercising regularly
- Drinking alcohol in moderation
- Getting enough sleep (minimum of seven hours a night)
- Trying to minimize stress (as we talked about in the first chapter)

Let's go into a couple of these in more detail.

Fruits and vegetables

As we've been discussing throughout the book, the food we eat is the single most important factor for determining health, and the resilience of our immune system is directly tied to what we're eating. We go into the specific foods suited to boosting immunity further in this chapter, but take note up front: Fruits and vegetables are extremely important, so make sure you're getting enough. Being proactive is important, so don't wait until you're sick. Drink one juice a day that consists mostly of green leafy vegetables and you'll enjoy the benefits of a stronger immune system.

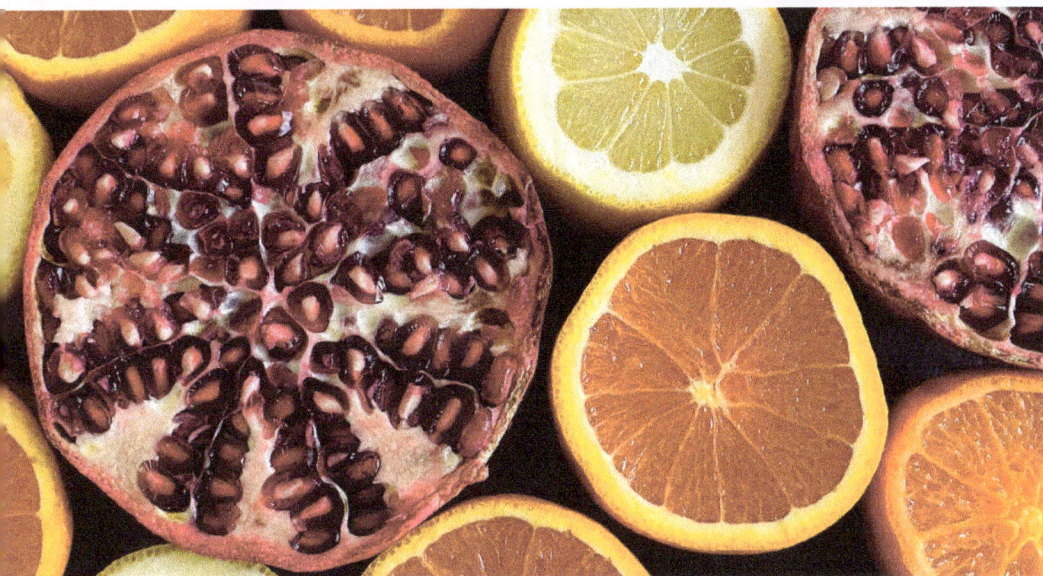

Regular exercise

Exercise is one of the pillars of healthy living. It strengthens your immune system by rejuvenating your cells and boosting your body's ability to fight off illness. Your heart, lungs, and muscles are all made stronger by exercise. It improves cardiovascular health, lowers blood pressure, helps control body weight, and protects against a variety of diseases. It may contribute even more directly by promoting good circulation, which allows the cells and substances of the immune system to move through the body freely. Try exercising six days a week for a minimum of twenty minutes.

Sleep

You should also prioritize sleep. During sleep, your immune system releases proteins called cytokines, some of which help promote good-quality sleep. Certain cytokines need to increase when you have an infection or inflammation, or when you're under stress. Sleep deprivation may decrease the production of these protective cytokines. In addition, infection-fighting antibodies and cells are reduced during periods when you don't get enough sleep.

Stress and immune function

Modern medicine is looking at the mind and body connection. As I've mentioned, the term 'fight or flight' is known as the stress response. It's what the body does as it prepares to confront or avoid danger. The stress response helps us rise to many challenges. But trouble starts when this response is constantly pro-voked by day-to-day events. Scientists are actively studying the relationship between stress and the immune system. The stress response suppresses the immune system, increasing susceptibility to colds and other illnesses

This was certainly Lisa's experience. Lisa is a wellness educator and transformational coach whose story shows how severe the effects of stress can be on your life and your health, and how the guidance you've read here can contribute to bringing you back to wellness.

LISA'S STORY

Life loves to throw curveballs, doesn't it? In my experi-ence, much-needed changes often start as gentle whispers, like, 'Take care of yourself, don't work so hard, eat better, do more of what you love,' but when we continue to ignore them, the whispers become louder, often becoming shouts, shoves, and, sometimes, if we really refuse to listen, life will bite us in unexpected places.

In February 2016, I was attempting to enjoy the last three months of a one-year, unpaid leave of absence from my demanding HR career with one of Canada's top-tier employers. Juggling the 'always on' 24/7 mentality at work and busy family life, which included managing complex special needs and caring responsibilities, had caused me to feel overwhelmed and exhausted. There simply wasn't enough of me to go around and I felt like I was falling short with everything and everyone. Chronic low-grade stress had been present in my life for many years and was show-ing up in my health in the form of insomnia, irritability, fatigue, regular bouts of strep throat, and finally, a brutal case of pneumonia that put me in bed for three weeks.

Instead of investing in burn-out recovery and self-discovery with a qualified coach or therapist, I directed all my attention and energy into 'fixing' everything and everyone around me, including all my family members and friends. I did not know how to be still and without the security of my prestigious business card and paycheck; I found myself bumping up against debilitating feelings of unworthiness and the vicious voice of my inner critic. I made myself even busier, picking up a couple of holistic nutrition courses and a yoga class to make my doctor happy, but my internal dialogue didn't change, and I remained entangled in life and workplace drama.

I received a literal 'bite' from life (god, the universe or whatever higher power has meaning for you) in the form of an infection and life-changing health crisis which forced me to finally wake up and change the way I eat, live, work and value myself. It happened during an unplanned visit to Australia.

While it would take five months to discover this, I was bitten by a sandfly carrying the Bartonella Henselae bacteria (more commonly known as cat scratch disease), who responded to my call for help by sharing a debilitating infection. On my return home to Canada and over the next few weeks and months, my body slowly shut down, initially manifesting as debilitating flu, followed by chronic inflammation, severe muscle pain to the point that I couldn't pick up a coffee cup, fatigue, brain fog, forgetfulness and eventually autoimmune disease. I could no longer not take notice of my escalating health situation or my long-term disconnection from the version of myself who dreamed, created, spoke up for myself and others, had fun, played, and believed that my gifts and knowledge could make a meaningful impact in the world. who was that person and how could I find her? I had become everything that I'd promised never to become: a sad, miserable, beaten-down, frustrated, unfulfilled forty-five-year-old who hated her job, barely saw her precious family, and didn't know how to prioritize her own needs.

By the time an April work deadline rolled around, I was so sick that I could barely get out of bed for more than a couple of hours a day. There was no way that I could return to a demanding senior management role, so while I had my way out, this was a far cry from the vision I had for my life. Now I was terribly ill, completely dependent on my husband for our finances and day-to-day support with the children and home duties, and I had no answers.

At that time, I had no idea why I was so sick or how to get better and I was terrified. It would take another few months of escalating symptoms before I finally got to see an infectious disease specialist and received a diagnosis to confirm that I had cat scratch disease. even though I'd never heard of it and had no idea how I could possibly have contracted it, I was hugely relieved that I wasn't 'only just' having a breakdown (as suggested by one particularly uncompassionate walk-in clinic doctor when I attempted to explain the pain and swelling in my arms and how I believed there was something wrong with my brain). The infection had gone to my brain and was causing me to lose words and I felt totally incompetent.

We started piecing together a treatment plan, but my immune system was in such poor shape that I required a three-month course of antibiotics. This killed the infection, but also knocked out all the healthy gut flora I had left. The severe inflammation, pain, and fatigue didn't go away, even months after results proved that I was no longer testing positive for the disease. The severity of the infection and my overstressed emotional state had created the optimal environment to trigger autoimmune disease. I had lost twenty pounds and was a walking skeleton.

What pained me was the knowledge that it all could have been avoided with effective self-care practices, diet, stress management and honoring who I was authentically. I resolved that if I'd created the conditions for disease, then I had the power to reverse it and reclaim my health.

When I think back to that time of illness, I feel immense gratitude to be on the other side of those debilitating and demoralizing symptoms, for the lessons learned and the love and encouragement from my husband, children, and friends like Lotus. I was fortunate to find a team of holistic healthcare professionals who helped me create a plan that included a strict anti-inflammatory diet, effective stress-management practices, daily meditation, and gentle movement, including yoga and Qi gong. It was a tough adjustment, but I wanted my life back and I was willing to do anything. I was finally ready to change.

Foods to help boost the immune system

A good immune system starts in the stomach. It needs good, regular nourishment. Scientists have recognized that people who live in poverty and are malnourished are more vulnerable to infectious diseases. There is evidence that various deficiencies of zinc, selenium, iron, copper, folic acid, and vitamins A, B, C, D, and E may increase the risk of a weakened immune system. While no one food or supplement can 'cure' or prevent you from catching a virus or the flu, some foods have been shown to help bolster immunity. Try to incorporate these ingredients into your regular eating routine.

Turmeric — This root has been shown to boost immune cell activity and enhance antibody responses, and it also contains an anti-inflammatory compound. Its health properties are thanks to curcumin, which also maintains a healthy cell cycle, enhances antioxidants, supports the body's natural detoxification system, and promotes healthy colon function.

Cayenne pepper – This spice used in soups, chilies, and curries will turn up the heat while it does its job eradicating bacteria and flu viruses before they start. An existing cold can also benefit from cayenne. Mix it in water with lemon to calm your cough and break up chest congestion.

Ginger – This has anti-inflammatory and antioxidative properties and offers many health benefits. Normal metabolic processes in the body, infections, and toxins all contribute to the production of free radicals, resulting in oxidative stress. Antioxidant compounds in ginger root have potent anti-inflammatory and immune-boosting properties.

Cinnamon – This spice has a long history of medicinal use when it comes to treating stomach upset, stomach flu, nausea, and stubborn colds due to its natural antibacterial and antiviral properties.

Garlic – This has antibacterial, antiviral, and antifungal properties. The bulbs are rich in antioxidants that quench the free radicals that play a role in heart disease, cancers, and other conditions. The antiviral properties may be helpful in reducing the severity of colds, flu, or other infections. Garlic contains allicin, a chemical compound that's been administered for centuries as a natural medicine to help ward off all sorts of flu viruses, fungi, and bacterial infections.

Citrus – Citrus fruits like oranges are an excellent source of vitamin C, which is the vitamin that many people turn to when they feel a cold developing. Vitamin C helps reduce the duration of common cold symptoms and improve the function of the human immune system.

Dry tart cherries – These support healthy sleep due to their natural melatonin content. This is crucial because research shows that people who don't get enough quality sleep are more likely to get sick after being exposed to a virus.

Pomegranates – This nutrient-dense superfood is another food that supports immunity via its antimicrobial and anti-inflammatory activity. The flavonoid antioxidants found in pomegranate juice have also been shown to decrease the length of a cold. Add pomegranate seeds to fruit salad or add splashes of juice to water or tea.

Elderberry – This has antiviral, anticancer, and anti-inflammatory properties. Elderberry is also high in flavonoids. People take elderberry supplements or tea as a remedy for colds, cases of flu, and bacterial sinus infections. Plant medicine works by reducing swelling in mucous membranes. Some studies suggest elderberry extract reduces the duration of the flu. If it works for flu infections, it may help your immune system against other infections.

Acai berry – This is such a potent antioxidant and stimulator of the immune system; researchers are studying it as a potential treatment for all kinds of conditions. The fruit is high in anthocyanins, flavonoid molecules that are very potent antioxidants. They combat oxidative stress in the body by mopping up free radicals. Antioxidants are credited with boosting immunity and lowering inflammation in the body.

Blueberries – This fruit contains a type of flavonoid called anthocyanin, which has antioxidant properties that can help boost a person's immune system. In addition, blueberries have plenty of vitamins and minerals, including vitamin C, vitamin A, potassium and manganese, and dietary fiber.

Root vegetables – Vegetables such as sweet potatoes, wild yams, jicama, beets, turnips, and parsnips are packed with soluble fiber that your gut loves and finds easy to digest. Carrots and sweet potatoes are wonderful sources of beta-carotene, a precursor to vitamin A. This nutrient aids the immune system by helping to produce white blood cells, which fight bacteria and viruses. It also helps form the mucous membranes that line the respiratory tract, which acts as a protective barrier to keep germs out of the body.

Pumpkin and squash — These vegetables are members of the Cucurbitaccac family and are the perfect immune system strengthener. Nutritionally, they have fiber, potassium, vitamin C, zinc, magnesium, manganese, and some B vitamins, like folate. Zinc influences multiple aspects of the immune system. As antioxidants, alpha- and beta-carotene and related phytonutrients (like lutein and zeaxanthin) are important for protecting body tissues from damage. They are incredibly helpful for protecting tissues and are promoted for a reduced risk of certain cancers. Pumpkin seeds are high in potassium, magnesium, iron, and copper. Try roasting the seeds! Pumpkin seeds are also a rich source of protein and the essential fatty acid omega-3.

Leafy green veggies — Leafy greens such as spinach provide anti-inflammatory antioxidants, as well as key nutrients known to help the immune system function, thanks to their high content of folate, vitamin A, vitamin C, fiber, magnesium, and iron. The nutrients boost immune function and provide the body with necessary nutrients for cell division and DNA repair. They also provide bioactive compounds that release a chemical signal that boosts immunity in the gut.

Cruciferous vegetables — This family of vegetables includes broccoli, cauliflower, Brussels sprouts, bok choy, arugula, radishes, watercress, and kale. They are anti-inflammatory superfoods high in many important nutrients. They also contain potent antioxidants, such as sulforaphane, a compound that may boost the production of glutathione. In terms of immune support, glutathione works by attacking free radicals to minimize their potential damage.

Mushrooms — Edible mushrooms contain powerful compounds that enhance your body's ability to fight diseases. Fungi are packed with antioxidants and anti-inflammatory components that destroy infections, slow down aging and regenerate nerve cells. These natural, protective ingredients work together to fight cancer, viruses, and inflammation to super-charge your immune system. They modify cytokines, which are inflammatory messengers that can suppress white blood cells and make you more susceptible to getting sick. Further, the polysaccharides that mushrooms are rich in help bolster and maintain the structure of your cells (essential in having a healthy immune system).

Sea vegetables – Seaweed keeps your sushi together, but it's not the only sea plant in the ocean that has major health benefits. Sea veggies are a source of protein, omega-3, chlorophyll, and dietary fiber, sodium, potassium, calcium, phosphorus, magnesium, iron, and other trace minerals naturally found in the ocean. Other varieties include dulse, nori, wakame, agar, arame, sea palm, spirulina and kombu. Edible seaweeds have long been a staple in Asian cultures.

Walnuts – In addition to being one of the top anti-inflammatory foods, walnuts contain several nutrients that play a role in supporting the immune system, including vitamins E and B6, copper and folate, and omega-3.

Almonds – These nuts are particularly high in vitamin E. In addition to vitamin C, vitamin E plays a key role in immunity. This fat-soluble vitamin boosts the activity of immune cells to support the body's ability to fend off bacteria and viruses.

Brazil nuts – These nuts contain a mineral called selenium, which enhances immunity. Selenium is also a potent antioxidant; it prevents cells from being attacked in ways that damage DNA. One ounce of brazil nuts, about six to eight whole nuts, provides nearly 1,000 percent of the daily value for selenium.

Salmon and other fish – Doctors, dietitians, and health experts all seem to agree omega-3 fatty acids is vitally essential to our overall health. Studies have shown that omega-3 can offer a vast array of health benefits ranging from joint health to memory. Oily fish are a great source of omega-3, which helps to boost the immune system by enhancing the functioning of immune cells. DHA-rich fish oil enhances the activity of white blood cells known as B cells. The popularity had led to hundreds of supplements flooding the marketplace. However, many contain impurities, diluted oils, and unwanted fillers. Try picking a good supplement or try plant based options like Seaweed, algae, hemp, walnuts, and chia seeds are also a good vegan source of omega-3.

Miso – Miso is a salty paste made from fermented soybeans. It is rich in probiotics that are beneficial for gastrointestinal (GI) health and boosting the immune system. A lack of beneficial bacteria or an imbalance of bacteria in the GI tract is associated with a variety of medical conditions. Beneficial microorganisms found in miso and other fermented foods perform a variety of necessary functions in the GI tract. The probiotics establish a healthy balance of flora in the GI tract, protecting against pathogenic strains that try to take hold. About seventy percent of the immune system lies in the gut. Healthy, balanced gut flora makes for a strong immune system.

Kefir and yogurt – These are fermented with live cultures of bacteria that are beneficial for health and boosting the immune system, fighting bad bacteria, and reducing inflammation. They can be made with dairy and you can now find dairy-free probiotic fermented coconut milk, which contains about two billion probiotic live cultures. Simply add to your smoothie!

Green tea – Green Tea is loaded with polyphenol antioxidants that have many health benefits, which include: Improved brain function, fat loss, protection against cancer and lowering heart disease. There may be more potential health benefits. Matcha Tea has exploded in popularity lately. Like green tea, matcha comes from the Camellia sinensis plant. The leaves are harvested and ground up into fine powder known as matcha. Matcha contains the nutrients from the entire leaf, which results in a greater amount of antioxidants than typically found in green tea.

Dark chocolate – This contains an antioxidant called theobromine, which helps to boost the immune system by protecting the body's cells from free radicals. Despite its potential benefits, dark chocolate is high in calories and saturated fat, so it is important to eat it in moderation.

First line of defense

Your first, and most important, line of defense against getting sick is your lifestyle. Not smoking or drinking heavily, making sure you exercise and get enough sleep, and choosing healthy foods will give you the best shot at reducing your chances of getting sick and minimizing the severity of an illness if you do.

CHAPTER 4

How to Care for Your Biggest Organ

'Nature gives you the face you have at twenty;
it is up to you to merit the face you have at fifty.'

COCO CHANEL

No, guys, I'm talking about skin! Did you know that skin is your biggest organ? Proper treatment can revitalize skin and slow the aging process, keeping skin healthier longer. Healthy skin isn't just important for looks — it's a passageway to our bloodstream, and the first barrier when it comes to fighting illness and diseases.

Your skin comprises two layers: the epidermis (outer) and the dermis (inner). It absorbs a large percentage of what you put on it. Be very careful you're not moisturizing your skin with chemical-laden lotions or scrubbing your body with toxic ingredients. Potentially dangerous chemicals can be found in your home. Household cleaning products can cause minor to serious problems and even life-threatening health problems.

Replace household cleaners and beauty products that are full of chemicals with organic and natural ones. You'll find health food stores are packed with these products or you could try making your own. Switching to homemade DIY cleaners and beauty products might sound like a lot more work, but it's actually quite simple and very inexpensive. The ingredients are easy to come by and last a long time.

Some of the ingredients in beauty products aren't that pretty. US researchers report that one in eight of the 82,000 ingredients used in personal care products are industrial chemicals, including carcinogens, pesticides, reproductive toxins, and hormone disruptors. Many products include plasticizers (chemicals that keep concrete soft), degreasers (used to get the grime off auto parts), and surfactants (which reduce surface tension in water, like in paint and inks). Imagine what that does to your skin, and to the environment.

Queen of Green surveyed Canadians to see how many of the 'Dirty Dozen' ingredients below appeared in their cosmetics, and the findings showed that eighty percent of entered products contained at least one of these toxic chemicals. You can avoid harmful chemicals by doing an audit of your cupboard using this list of harmful ingredients:

1. BHA and BHT
2. Coal tar dyes: p-phenylenediamine and colors listed as 'CI'
3. DEA-related ingredients
4. Dibutyl phthalate
5. Formaldehyde-releasing preservatives
6. Parabens
7. Perfume (a.k.a. fragrance)
8. PEG compounds
9. Petrolatum
10. Siloxanes
11. Sodium laureth sulfate
12. Triclosan

Another resource is a wonderful site called Cosmetic Database: www. ewg.org/skindeep. This non-profit site is run by the Environmental Working Group (EWG), whose staff scientists take the ingredients found in more than 75,000 popular health and beauty products and cross-reference them with information found in more than sixty toxicity and regulatory databases. EWG then comes up with a 0-10 safety rating for each product and provides links between individual ingredients and studies that have proven possible organ toxicity, reproductive issues, or carcinogenic effects.

To use the site, simply type in the name of your product and you'll be redirected to a product page that lists each ingredient, along with any potential health concerns and a score between 0 and10. A score of 0 indicates a pretty innocuous product with little to no proven health concerns, while a score of 10 indicates something you most likely do not want to be slathering all over your skin any time soon. It's one way to educate yourself about the products you're using, and also a great way to demystify the process of buying 'safe' products.

Ingredients for healthy skin and home

The below are the best DIY ingredients for potent and effective potions. When it comes to making your own DIY skincare and household cleaning products, the idea is to have some fun and get creative. You'll find DIY recipes at the end of the chapter, but let's look first at the benefits of the substances involved.

Aloe vera – Not only is aloe vera great at healing sunburn, but it contains bacteria-fighting, soothing ingredients that fight inflammation, redness, and itching. It also has antimicrobial and antifungal properties, making it great as a hydrating facial scrub. Squirt a nice-sized dollop into clean hands and scrub your face gently, washing with warm water.

Sea salt – Sea salt comes loaded with tons of minerals and nutrients like calcium, magnesium, and potassium. Salt helps pores balance oil production, reduces inflammation, fights off bacteria, and brightens skin. Use sea salt in homemade scrubs and bath salts. It can be mixed with ingredients like coconut oil and essential oils. This **salt contains anti-inflammatory properties** which soothe skin and calm breakouts.

Epsom salts — These are used to soften skin and exfoliate. Epsom salts are a source of magnesium, which has been shown to ease stress, lower blood pressure and create a happy and relaxed feeling. It's best to buy it unscented and simply add a few drops of your favorite 100 percent natural essential oils to your Epsom salts bath.

Oatmeal — This is very moisturizing. Use to relieve itchiness and dry skin. Grind the oatmeal before adding to bathwater. You can use regular store-bought oatmeal or a holistic powder type.

Lemon juice — Lemons are a great all-purpose odor remover in the kitchen and useful for removing stains. Run half a lemon over a dirty cutting board to help remove odors such as onion or fish. Put half a lemon down the disposal (chop it up if your disposal has trouble with large objects) and grind it to remove odors from the kitchen sink. Lemon juice adds cleaning power to all-purpose solutions.

Baking soda — Also known as sodium bicarbonate, this is a kitchen staple, but it can also be used in beauty products. Use baking soda for scrubbing, to eliminate odors, and to whiten. You can even use baking soda to whiten your teeth.

Hydrogen peroxide — This is a powerful disinfectant for killing mildew. Combine with baking soda to create a paste, put it on the mildew and allow to sit for a few minutes before wiping away. This paste can be used to whiten clothes too.

Vinegar — This is a powerhouse of cleaning. When disinfecting and deodorizing, vinegar is a go-to product for spots on countertops (though not recommended for marble surfaces). Apple cider vinegar is also wonderful in DIY beauty care recipes.

Essential oils

For over 5,000 years, many different cultures have used healing plant oils for a variety of health conditions. Whether used for relaxation, beauty care, home cleaning, or as natural remedies, essential oils carry the pure power of the plant.

As the essential oil market continues to grow, many consumers are unaware of the potential risks of using essential oils in their wellness, beauty, and cleaning routines. Whether a specific oil is safe for you depends on a number of factors. When it comes to the oil, it's important to consider the chemical composition and purity, method of use, and dosage.

Although essential oils are presumed to be chemical-free, it's always best to read the labels to know what you're buying. Pure essential oils are strong, so you only need a small amount. Always do a sniff test before buying to make sure you're not sensitive to the fumes and use caution when handling them. A few drops of essential oil can add antibacterial and antifungal power to a cleaning solution. Add a few drops of your favorite essential oil to your bath and help calm the mind and body.

Lavender oil – Lavender has a very pleasant aroma and is very relaxing. A few drops on your pillow can ensure sound sleep. It is not a bad idea to use it in your bathwater, too, to increase its calming effect. It's also a very potent antiseptic and works well to help heal cuts and bruises.

Rose oil – A delicate fragrance oil, rose oil is known to calm and moisturize skin. It can be used in natural beauty treatments to improve acne and balance hormones. Rose essential oil may help to release stress, improve the quality of your sleep and benefit women undergoing menopause.

Lemon oil – Lemon oil has a variety of uses and benefits. With a clean, fresh, citrus aroma, lemon is known for its purifying properties. Often used in cleaning products, lemon has distinct cleansing and deodorizing characteristics. As a versatile oil, lemon also has the ability to aid in digestion and support healthy respiratory function when taken internally. Whether it is being diffused, taken internally, or applied topically, lemon oil is a good remedy for restoring the luster of dull skin. It is astringent and detoxifying in nature. Its antiseptic properties help in treating pimples and various other skin disorders. Lemon is also recommended for reducing excessive oil on the skin. It can make your skin photosensitive when applied topically, so only use a few drops of this essential oil combined with a good carrier oil (discussed below).

Sweet orange oil – Sweet orange reduces anxiety and may uplift your mood when inhaled. It boosts the immune system, prevents infection, and reduces inflammation. Lemon and orange are wonderful disinfectants. Like lemon oil, this oil can make your skin photosensitive when applied topically, so only use a few drops of this essential oil combined with a good carrier oil.

Chamomile oil – Chamomile essential oil can help you get rid of skin blemishes, acne, and inflammation. This oil also works perfectly with coconut oil to lessen the effects of diaper rash. Chamomile is an effective stress reliever and can help you get a good night's sleep.

Peppermint oil – Peppermint produces a pleasant, cooling, and calming sensation when applied topically, and it can help reduce skin inflammation. This oil can help stimulate blood circulation, your scalp, and hair follicles. It can also help alleviate headaches and congestion and relieve digestive issues.

Frankincense oil – Frankincense essential oil has an aroma that is relaxing. It is commonly used in the East before yoga sessions and meditation. It greatly reduces stress and depression and increases spiritual awareness. It is also a perfect antiseptic that helps minor cuts and insect bites heal. It is ideal for fungal infections on your skin and is usually an ingredient in natural shampoo to help get rid of dandruff.

Eucalyptus – This smells like Vicks Vaporub or Tiger Balm. Eucalyptus is a popular ingredient in balm, massage blends, and inhalers. It supports the respiratory system and aids decongestion. With its antiseptic qualities, it has the ability to kill fungus, bacteria, and even parasites. It can boost your immune system and is anti-inflammatory.

Tea tree oil – Tea tree fights breakouts, redness, and inflammation on the skin. It's antibacterial, antimicrobial, and antifungal as well as anti-inflammatory. In Australia, essential oil has been around for over a century. Tea tree oil is one of the best home remedies for acne and is also wonderful as a cleaning agent.

Oregano oil – This oil benefits many homemade cleaners. Due to oregano's chemical makeup, it's a powerful cleanser and purifying agent. Mix a few drops in a spray bottle with water to clean surfaces and countertops, even natural stone. This oil is also a natural antibiotic, which helps support the immune system and respiratory function and may improve gut health.

Rosemary oil – Invigorating. Refreshing. Stimulating. These are the first three words that come to mind. Rosemary is helpful in massage and arthritis blends and can help improve circulation. It is useful for respiratory issues and makes a good expectorant/decongestant. Rosemary has an excellent reputation for helping with oily skin/acne, scalp, and hair care. Rosemary is quite stimulating and is lauded for aiding memory retention and staying focused and alert.

Carrier oils

Carrier oils, also known as base oils, dilute the concentration of essential oils before they are applied and carry the essential oil into the skin. Carrier oils are used in aromatherapy, a therapy where various essential oils are applied to the body to aid both physical and emotional wellbeing.

Almond oil – Not only does almond oil smell great, but it also has anti-inflammatory, antiviral, antibacterial, and antiseptic properties. It makes a great carrier oil for essential oils for rashes, acne, or dryness.

Olive oil – Olive oil can naturally condition wood, as well as skin and hair! Packed with anti-aging antioxidants and hydrating squalene, this makes it superb for hair, skin, and nails. Just like coconut oil, it's essential in any DIY beauty kit. It has been used as a hair treatment since ancient Egyptian times.

Avocado oil – Avocado oil contains vitamins A, D, and E, which are able to penetrate the skin. It helps soothe sunburned skin, can boost collagen production, and treats age spots. It also works to reduce inflammation of the skin when applied topically and can do the same internally when eaten.

Coconut oil – This oil can be used on skin and hair. It strengthens the epidermal tissue, removing dead skin cells, and can help protect us from sunburn. Containing antibacterial, antiviral, antifungal, and antioxidant properties, it also helps cleanse, moisturize, heal wounds and prevent razor burn.

Argan oil – Native to Morocco, this oil is so healing because it's rich in vitamin A and vitamin E, various antioxidants, and omega fatty acids, including linoleic acid. Argan is great for gently moisturizing skin and giving you healthy hair.

Shea butter – Around for hundreds of years, shea butter is an excellent moisturizing option for dry skin types and is inexpensive yet effective at reducing flaking, redness, or peeling. Great for making lip balms if you just add a little essential oil.

Jojoba oil – Native to the southern US and Mexico, this oil is used to treat acne, psoriasis, sunburn, dry skin, and wrinkles. It's also used to reduce balding because it encourages hair regrowth, soothes the skin, and unclogs hair follicles. When it comes to the chemical structure of jojoba oil, it's unique in that it's a polyunsaturated wax.

Rosehip oil – Harvested from the seeds of rose bushes, this powerhouse is packed with anti-inflammatory fatty acids, antioxidants, and vitamins A and C. It does wonderful things for your face.

Natural solutions – inside and out

Do-it-yourself beauty products are a huge trend right now. It's a great way to save money and avoid the toxins in commercial beauty products. I invite you to be a chemist and try developing some of your own potions and lotions with the natural ingredients I mentioned above. There are some recipes to try in the next section. If you go online, you'll find many websites like lolaessentials. biz where you can learn more about essential oils and what you can do with them.

While the natural ingredients we've been discussing can be very effective for healing skin and promoting good health, what you put into your body also plays an enormous role in your outer appearance. A healthy diet, good sleep, exercise, and drinking plenty of water really can improve someone's looks. Certain supplements can also help improve the effectiveness of your beauty regime. Let's talk about the natural elements you can consume to help take care of your skin.

Water – Water flushes toxins out and allows your body to experience a 'detox'. Removing things like bacteria and waste from your system stops them from affecting your skin. Of course, water plays a big role in keeping skin hydrated and looking young. Most experts recommend drinking at least eight glasses of plain water every single day. Did you know that water makes up about seventy percent of your body?

Is the water you're drinking clean? Pharmaceuticals, treated sewage, disinfectants, agricultural runoff, industrial waste, and other chemicals can be found in drinking water these days. Municipal water systems compound these issues by treating water with chlorine and similar chemicals. If you are using well water, fertilizers, pesticides, and bacteria, as well as calcium and magnesium, can leech into the water. I recommend getting a filtration system to purify your drinking water.

Collagen protein – Collagen helps build healthy skin cells and is partially responsible for skin's youthful elasticity, softness, and firmness. It also helps prevent joint pain, reduces inflammation, improves gut health, and stimulates nail and hair growth. While many topical products add collagen to their formula to boost its appeal, it's actually much more effective when taken internally. Marine collagen, which is type 1 collagen, is made of peptides derived from fish and has the most efficient absorption of all collagen types. When considering supplements, you should look for a high quality source. Such as wild caught marine collagen or grass fed bovine collagen peptide supplement.

Probiotics – Probiotics are the 'good' bacteria that help balance our gut environment. They are tied to improved immunity, helping your immune and nervous system deal with toxins like bad bacteria, yeast, viruses, fungi, and parasites, all of which can show up on your skin.

Prebiotics – Prebiotics, like chicory root fiber, are derived from plants that belong to the dandelion family and are primarily composed of inulin. They have been linked to improved blood sugar control and digestive health, among other health benefits.

Vitamin B complex – Vitamin B helps prevent infections and supports cell health, growth of red blood cells, healthy brain function, good digestion, energy levels, proper nerve function, and good eyesight.

Omega-3 – Omega-3s are loaded with healthy fatty acids that help keep skin moisturized and elastic. They also help regulate hormone function, nervous system health, and immune function.

Foods have a big impact on the condition of your skin. If you still suffer from acne and frequent skin problems, eat lots of leafy greens and consider doing an elimination diet by cutting out sugar, dairy, and gluten. Many people are intolerant or allergic to dairy and/or gluten (wheat, barley, and rye) and this can manifest in skin issues.

It's worth noting that stress and a lack of sleep can be the cause of a hormonal imbalance that leads to skin breakouts. Beauty sleep is more than just a silly saying. Not getting good sleep has an effect on the body similar to stress. Both stress and lack of sleep make your body conserve energy, which compromises skin health. During sleep, your skin's blood flow increases, and the organs rebuild collagen, repairing damage from UV exposure, and reducing wrinkles and age spots.

DIY skincare

Start with a basic blend of carrier oils like the ones listed earlier, then add a few drops of essential oils to help enhance the benefits of your anti-aging natural skincare cleansers, masks, and serums. When using essential oils in skincare blends, less is best! Normal dilution is 2.5 percent, or ten drops of essential oil to two tablespoons of carrier oil.

FACIAL SERUM FOR DRY SKIN

2 tablespoons avocado oil
1 tablespoon jojoba oil
1 tablespoon rosehip oil
6 drops lavender essential oil

Add the carrier oils to a dark glass bottle. Then add the essential oils and shake well. Apply 2 drops to the face and neck. Shake before each use.

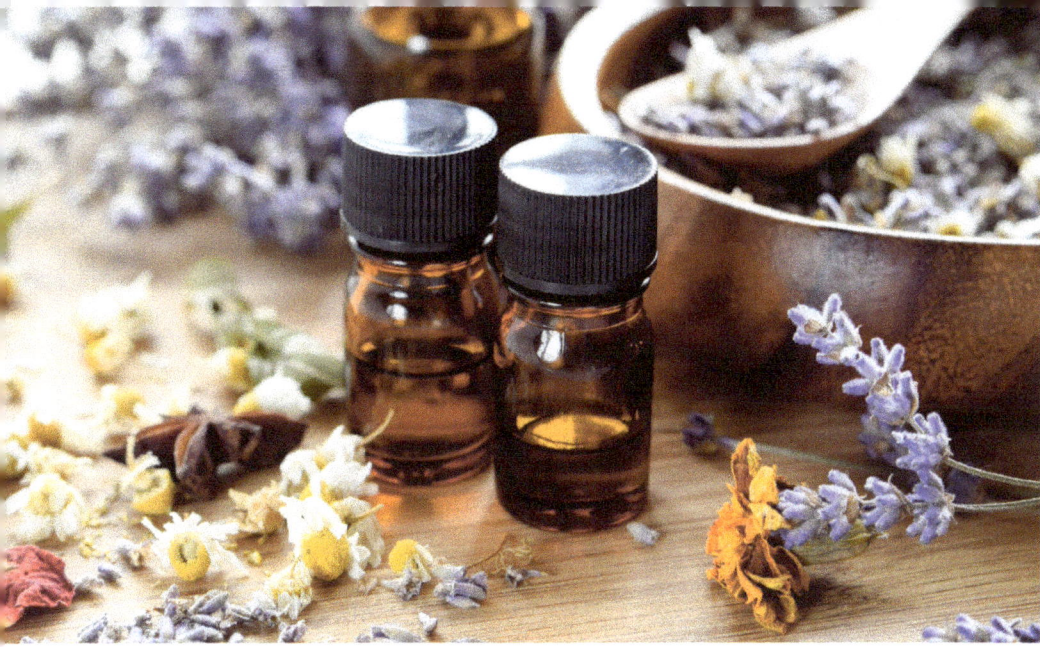

ALMOND OIL FACE SERUM

2 tablespoons almond oil
5 drops frankincense essential oil
3 drops chamomile essential oil
2 drops lavender essential oil
3 drops rosehip essential oil

Add the carrier oils to a dark glass bottle. Then add the essential oils and shake well. Apply 2 drops to the face and neck. Shake before each use.

GENTLE OATMEAL FACE CLEANSER

½ cup ground oatmeal
2 tablespoons filtered water

Mix the oatmeal with enough water to form a paste. Smooth over the entire face, avoiding the eye area. Allow to sit for ten minutes and rinse.

EPSOM BODY EXFOLIATE

2 cups Epsom salt
¼ cup coconut oil
3 drops lavender essential oil

Mix ingredients. Use the mixture to gently scrub away dry skin patches.

ITCH-RELIEVER BATH SALTS

2 cups Epsom salts
1 cup sea salt or rock salt
2 tablespoons baking soda
3 drops chamomile essential oil
3 drops peppermint essential oil
3 drops lavender essential oil

Mix salts together in a bowl. Stir in the remaining ingredients. When using essential oils, add one drop at a time, stirring well. Allow mixture to dry completely for six hours before packaging. Store in glass jars.

BATH OIL

2 tablespoons base carrier oil
5 drops rose essential oil
5 drops lavender essential oil

Simply add the drops of oil directly to the bathtub or mix the oils in a dark glass bottle and save for future use.

DIY household cleaners

Cleaning your house naturally is not difficult or expensive. These homemade all-natural cleaning recipes will help you save money and minimize exposure to harsh toxins. They improve indoor air quality and are much safer, especially for children. Use these tips and recipes to clean your house.

ALL-PURPOSE CLEANER

Two-parts distilled water
One-part white vinegar
Essential oil (optional)

Add all ingredients to a spray bottle and shake to mix. For extra antibacterial and antifungal properties, add 20 drops of tea tree essential oil.

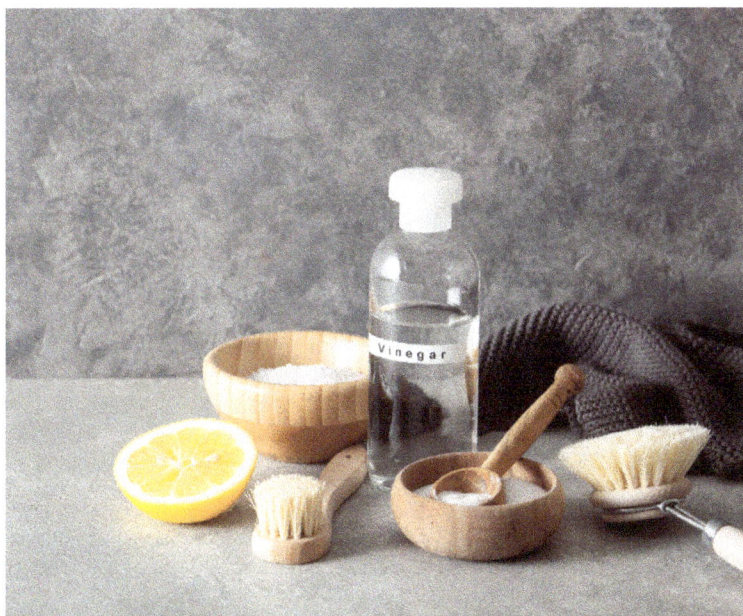

SCENTED ALL-PURPOSE CLEANER

Two-parts distilled water
One-part white vinegar
Lemon rind
Rosemary sprigs

Add all ingredients to a spray bottle and shake to mix. for extra cleaning power and an invigorating scent, add 15 drops of rosemary essential oil.

WOOD CLEANER

1½ cups distilled water
1 cup white vinegar
8 tablespoons olive oil
Lemon essential oil (optional)

Add all ingredients to a spray bottle and shake to mix. for extra cleaning power and a lively, fresh scent, add 20 drops of lemon essential oil.

TUB AND SHOWER CLEANER

One-part white vinegar
One-part natural dish soap
One-part distilled water

Using a funnel, add all ingredients to a spray bottle and shake to mix. For extra cleaning power and a lively, fresh scent, add 20 drops of lemon essential oil.

CARPET STAIN REMOVER

Baking soda (enough to cover the stain)
1 tablespoon natural liquid dishwasher soap
1 tablespoon white vinegar
2 cups warm water

Sprinkle the stain with the baking soda and let sit for fifteen minutes. Combine dish soap, vinegar, and water in a bowl. Sponge the mixture onto the stain and then blot using a dry cloth. Repeat until the stain disappears.

Read the labels

By reading labels and trying to limit harmful ingredients found in some skincare products and household cleaners, you'll be promoting detoxification and improving your health.

CHAPTER 5

What Causes Inflammation and How to Avoid It

'No disease that can be treated by diet should
be treated with any other means.'

MAIMONIDES

According to a study from Harvard University, inflammation is linked to most modern health conditions. Inflammation is actually the body's natural response to safeguard against foreign bacteria, viruses, and infection. It is part of the body's defense mechanism and plays a role in the healing process. When the body senses a threat such as an irritant, thorn, or pathogen, it will trigger the release of chemicals and white blood cells. Sometimes, however, the body mistakenly perceives its own cells or tissues as harmful. This reaction can lead to autoimmune diseases such as multiple sclerosis, rheumatoid arthritis or osteoarthritis, fibromyalgia, allergies, psoriasis, inflammatory bowel disease, celiac disease, Crohn's disease, colitis, type 1 diabetes, cardiovascular diseases, and many more.

I live my life by the 80/20 rule. Most days I exercise and eat a very healthy vegan diet. However, twenty percent of the time I might indulge in champagne, birthday cake or pizza, or skip a yoga class. Making healthy lifestyle choices most of the time without depriving yourself or feeling guilty about occasional indulgence is key. Life is meant to be lived and enjoyed.

I usually start my day off with green tea and cold-pressed juice with whatever vegetables I can find in my kitchen. However, the same is not true if I am on vacation in France. I would probably choose a croissant with a café au lait or a mimosa.

So, let's take a closer look at what foods we should be choosing eighty percent of the time, and why. These foods are the superfoods, which decrease inflammation and promote vitality. You'll notice crossover once more with the foods that boost immunity that we went through earlier in the book – it's great to know that if you're working to boost immunity via changes to your diet then you're also reducing your inflammation, and vice versa!

Anti-inflammatory food

These foods are proven to help reduce LDL cholesterol and blood pressure and improve brain health.

Omega-3 – What makes omega-3 fats special? They are an integral part of the cell membranes throughout the body and affect the function of the cell receptors in these membranes. They provide the starting point for making hormones that regulate blood clotting, contraction and relaxation of artery walls, and inflammation. Omega-3s are part of the polyunsaturated family. Marine omega-3 Docosahexaenoic acid (DHA) comes mainly from fish like salmon, mackerel, cod, herring, anchovies, caviar, and sardines. Alpha-linolenic acid (ALA) is found in vegetable oils and nuts (especially walnuts), flax, hemp, and chia seeds. Seaweed and algae are a great source of Omega-3 for people on a plant-based diet, as they are one of a few plant groups that contain DHA and EPA.

Nuts and seeds – Nuts such as walnuts, almonds, hazelnuts, and pistachios, and seeds such as flax, hemp, and chia are full of antioxidants that help protect against disease and reduce inflammation. When making your next salad, add a little crunch with a handful of nuts or seeds instead of croutons.

Complex whole grains – These contain a host of anti-inflammatory compounds, B vitamins, protein, and fiber. To take advantage of these, replace white rice with brown rice or quinoa in your favorite recipes.

Turmeric – This root is one of the most powerful and versatile anti-inflammatory foods. Its health properties are thanks to curcumin, which also maintains a healthy cell cycle, enhances antioxidants, supports the body's natural detoxification system, and promotes healthy colon function.

Ginger – This belongs to the Zingiberaceae family and is closely related to turmeric. With a long history of use in various forms of traditional /alternative medicine, it has been used to help digestion, reduce nausea and fight the common cold.

Garlic, onions, and leeks – These contain diallyl disulfides, an anti-inflammatory compound.

Asparagus – Asparagus is packed with fiber, folate, and other B vitamins. It has four grams of protein per eight stalks. It's a prebiotic and also a natural diuretic to beat bloating.

Dark leafy greens – These are high in vitamin E, an antioxidant with superior anti-inflammatory properties.

Cruciferous vegetables – This vegetable family includes cauliflower, kale, Brussels sprouts, cabbage, bok choy, and broccoli. These are anti-inflammatory superfoods high in many important nutrients.

Avocados – Packed with potassium, magnesium, fiber, and heart-healthy monounsaturated fats, avocadoes also contain carotenoids and tocopherols, which are linked to reduced cancer risk. They are high in vitamin E and monounsaturated fats, two anti-inflammatory powerhouses that help improve skin, joints, brain function, and cardiovascular health.

Root veggies – Roots such as sweet potatoes, wild yams, jicama, beets, carrots, turnips, and parsnips are packed with soluble fiber that your gut loves and finds easy to digest. Carrots and sweet potatoes in particular are rich in beta-carotene and vitamin A, which are believed to fight inflammation.

Mushrooms – Mushrooms are very low in calories and rich in selenium, copper, and all of the B vitamins. They also contain phenols and other antioxidants that provide anti-inflammatory protection. Thousands of varieties of mushrooms exist worldwide, but only a few are edible. These include truffles, portobello mushrooms, button mushrooms, and shitake. Chaga mushroom tea has a number of wonderful health benefits.

The Food and Drug Administration (FDA) recently approved the use of hallucinogenic active ingredient psilocybin founds in magic mushrooms to treat depression.

Cherries – These are delicious and rich in antioxidants, such as anthocyanins and catechins.

Grapes – These contain anthocyanins, which reduce inflammation. Grapes are also one of the best sources of resveratrol, another compound that has many health benefits.

Citrus fruit – Citrus fruits such as oranges, grapefruits, lemons, and limes are all rich in vitamin C, which is an important ingredient in tissue repair. They are also a good source of inflammation-fighting antioxidants.

Apples – These contain an antioxidant called quercetin as well as being a great source of fiber. An apple a day might just keep the doctor away, but their natural pectin fiber is the reason they're so great for your gut. Pectin feeds good bacteria and apples are also a good source of inulin and natural FOS (a beneficial type of sugar that feeds the gut). Apples are good for keeping you full and warding off high cholesterol. Choose Granny Smith if you're watching your sugar intake and always choose organic, since apples are high on the Dirty Dozen list of pesticide-laden fruits and veggies.

Pomegranates – This fruit is actually in the berry family. Pomegranates have an impressive nutrient profile and anti-inflammatory effect due to the antioxidant properties of the punicalagin.

Berries – Meanwhile, berries such as blueberries, raspberries, and blackberries are packed with fiber, vitamins, and minerals. They contain antioxidants called anthocyanins. These compounds may reduce inflammation, boost immunity and reduce your risk of heart disease.

Pineapple – Pineapple's key anti-inflammatory is bromelain, an enzyme that helps improve protein digestion.

Dark chocolate – As well as being delicious, rich, and satisfying, dark chocolate is also packed with antioxidants that reduce inflammation, reducing your risk of disease and leading to healthier aging.

Green tea – This is one of the healthiest beverages you can drink. Many of its benefits are due to its antioxidant and anti-inflammatory properties, especially a substance called epigallocatechin-3-gallate (EGCG), which inhibits inflammation by reducing pro-inflammatory cytokine production and damage to the fatty acids in your cells.

Red wine – While most famous for containing polyphenol, it's the resveratrol in red wine that is shown to prevent chronic systemic inflammation. Drink in moderation. Too much alcohol also causes inflammation, so try not to overdo it. It does not mix with certain medications so it's best to talk to your doctor if you are taking prescription drugs.

Extra virgin olive oil – This is one of the healthiest fats you can eat. It is rich in monounsaturated fats and a staple in the Mediterranean diet, which provides numerous health benefits. Anti-inflammatory benefits are much greater in extra virgin olive oil than in more refined olive oils.

Cannabidiol (CDB) oil – Studies have shown that CDB may help reduce chronic pain by impacting endocannabinoid receptor activity, reducing inflammation, and interacting with neurotransmitters. It can also alleviate cancer-related symptoms and side effects like nausea. Add a few drops to your morning smoothie.

Instructions for an anti-inflammatory diet

Anti-inflammatory foods are those that most nutrition experts would encourage you to eat. They include lots of fruits and vegetables, plant-based proteins (nuts, seeds, lentils, and beans), and lots of fresh herbs and spices. Eat fish rich in omega-3 if you are not vegan. Go for a variety of fruits and veggies. The greener the better!

Protein

Having small amounts of protein with every meal is key. The optimal serving size at any one sitting is the size of your palm. Here are some recommendations:

Fish – Unlimited. Choose fish that are sustainable and low in mercury. Stick to salmon, sardines, mackerel, trout, cod, and herring. Think small! Big fish that are higher up on the food chain eat smaller ones, which accumulate higher levels of mercury in their fat. For more information visit websites like www.fda.gov/food/consumers/advice-about-eating-fish which provides more recommendations.

Legumes - Unlimited. These foods combat inflammation because they're loaded with anti-inflammatory compounds, fiber and protein. Add more chickpeas and lentils to your diet. Some people are sensitive to legumes, which can cause an inflammatory response. Therefore, it is important to see how your body responds to lectins which are hard to break down. However, soaking, sprouting and cooking beans and legumes can neutralize the lectins.

Nuts and seeds – Limited. Nuts and seeds are rich in magnesium and vitamin E. Some are high omega-3 also. Ideally, you should reach for raw and unsalted. Nuts and seeds are high in calories, so don't eat them mindlessly. Walnuts, almonds, pumpkin, chia, and flax seeds are a staple in my house.

Eggs – Unlimited. Choose omega-3 enriched eggs (from hens that have been fed a flax meal diet) or organic eggs from free-range chickens when possible.

Dairy – None or limited - If you don't have a dairy intolerance you may have goat cheese or parmesan cheese if you have to eat dairy, because they have less lactose content, but please limit your intake).

Fruit

Fresh fruit – All fresh fruit is allowed. Emphasize those high in bio-flavonoids. Choose fruits from all parts of the color spectrum, especially berries and orange and yellow fruits. Choose organic when possible. Learn which conventionally grown foods are most likely to contain residual pesticide on page 25.

Dried fruit – Little to none. They are too high in sugar, so please limit.

Frozen fruit – Great for use in smoothies, frozen fruits and veggies can have just as many vitamins and nutrients compared to fresh.

Vegetables

Eat as many vegetables as you can with the exception of nightshade veggies (eggplant, peppers, tomatoes, and white potatoes). Increase intake of dark leafy greens, mushrooms, garlic, onions, leeks, ginger, and turmeric. Increase intake of cruciferous vegetables (broccoli, kale, Brussels sprouts, cabbage, etc.)

Green/dark leafy green veggies, red/yellow/orange vegetables – Unlimited.

White potatoes – None, but sweet potatoes are encouraged.

Grains

Limit to complex carbohydrates. The majority should be in the form of less refined, less processed foods which are lower on the glycemic index load. Reduce your consumption of foods made with wheat flour and sugar. You'll want to increase your fiber intake also.

Wheat or gluten (pasta or bread) – None.

Quinoa, brown rice, oat, buckwheat, millet, amaranth – Encouraged. Whole grains tend to be high in fiber and fiber also helps with inflammation.

Snacks

Seeds and nuts – These should be raw, not seasoned, and stored in the refrigerator to keep them fresh for longer and prevent them going rancid.

Nut butters – Use almond, cashew, hazelnut, etc.

Fresh fruit and veggies – Unlimited.

Beverages

Focus on water, and green or herbal tea.

Sweeteners

Refined sugar, corn syrup, high fructose corn syrup – None.

Stevia, honey, and maple syrup – Limited amounts if you must.

Oils

Avocado, sesame, and olive oil are the way to go.

Lotus's weekly shopping list

By following this shopping list, you can slowly and easily add anti-inflammatory foods to your diet.

Produce

- Bananas
- Apples
- Oranges
- Cherries
- Pomegranate
- Pineapple
- Avocado
- Lemons/limes
- Garlic
- Leafy greens
- Kale
- Asparagus
- Cabbage
- Mushrooms
- Beets
- Onions
- Carrots
- Jerusalem artichokes
- Sweet potato
- Squash
- Pumpkin
- Cucumber
- Broccoli
- Basil, cilantro, parsley, ginger root, turmeric, and other spices or herbs of your choice
- Any veggies you want in pasta, stir fry, or curry dish (fresh or frozen)
- Other fruits of your choice for snacking and fruit salad

Fridge/freezer

- Frozen organic blueberries (or other berries)
- Hummus (or make your own)
- Wild salmon fillets
- Wild fish of your choice
- Healthy gluten-free bread
- Pesto (or make your own – can be frozen)
- Nut-based vegan yogurt
- Coconut kefir
- Goat's cheese
- Parmesan cheese (a small amount goes a long way)

Canned and dry foods

- Brown rice or brown basmati rice
- Brown rice pasta
- Quinoa
- Brown rice crackers
- Nuts for snacks (unsalted almonds, cashews, etc.)
- Seeds for salads or cereal (sesame, pumpkin, flax, etc.)
- Gluten-free oatmeal
- Dry organic lentils
- Organic chickpeas
- Chia seeds
- Hemp hearts
- Seaweed
- Gluten-free granola or make your own (you'll find a recipe in the next part of the book!)

Pantry basics

- Olive, avocado, sesame, coconut, and nut oils
- Vegan protein powder and collagen powder for morning smoothies
- Organic raw honey, Stevia, or maple syrup
- Red wine, apple cider, balsamic vinegar

- Miso
- Tamari
- Coconut milk
- Vegetable or bone broth
- Almond or other non-dairy milk, unsweetened (or make your own)

Making healthier meals

The first part of the book has been about giving you the tools you need to succeed. By making a few simple modifications to your lifestyle, you can easily transform your body and mindset to rewrite your story. Simply by reading labels before you add items to your shopping carts. Choosing whole foods which will increase your good gut bacteria, boost your immunity, and lower inflammation. Learning to reduce cortisol (the stress hormone) by exercising regularly, practicing meditation, and getting enough sleep. All will help your body stay healthy.

It's important to be informed and understand the effects that not eating healthily and not getting enough sleep or exercise have on the body. It starts with one little step at a time to transform your life from surviving to thriving. If you need extra tips or help to stay on track, go to lotusfineliving.com or friend me on Facebook or Instagram.

Now that you have a better understanding of what all these different foods do to the body and why, let's address putting them all together in delicious recipes that you'll look forward to eating and drinking.

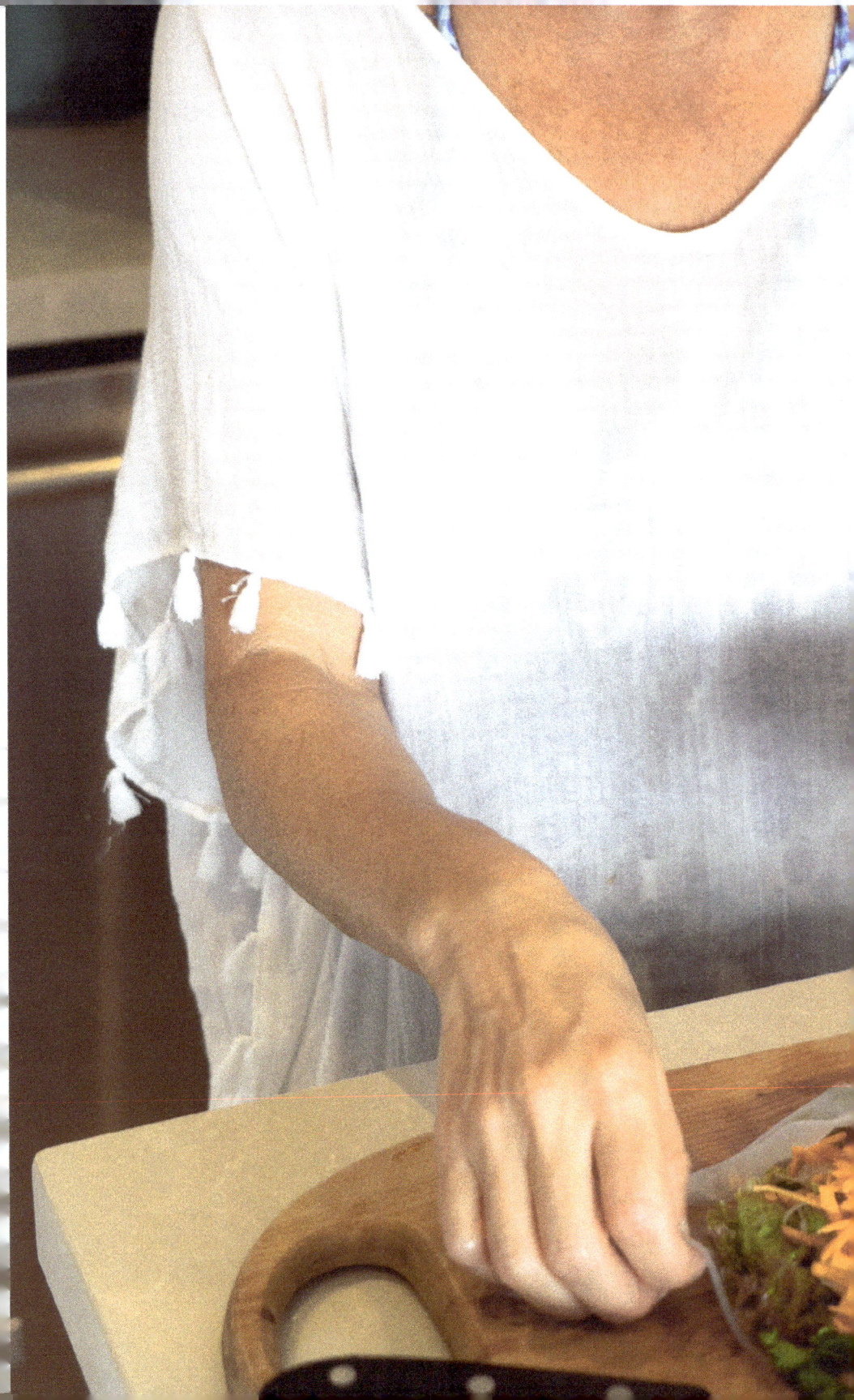

PART TWO

MAKING HEALTHIER MEALS

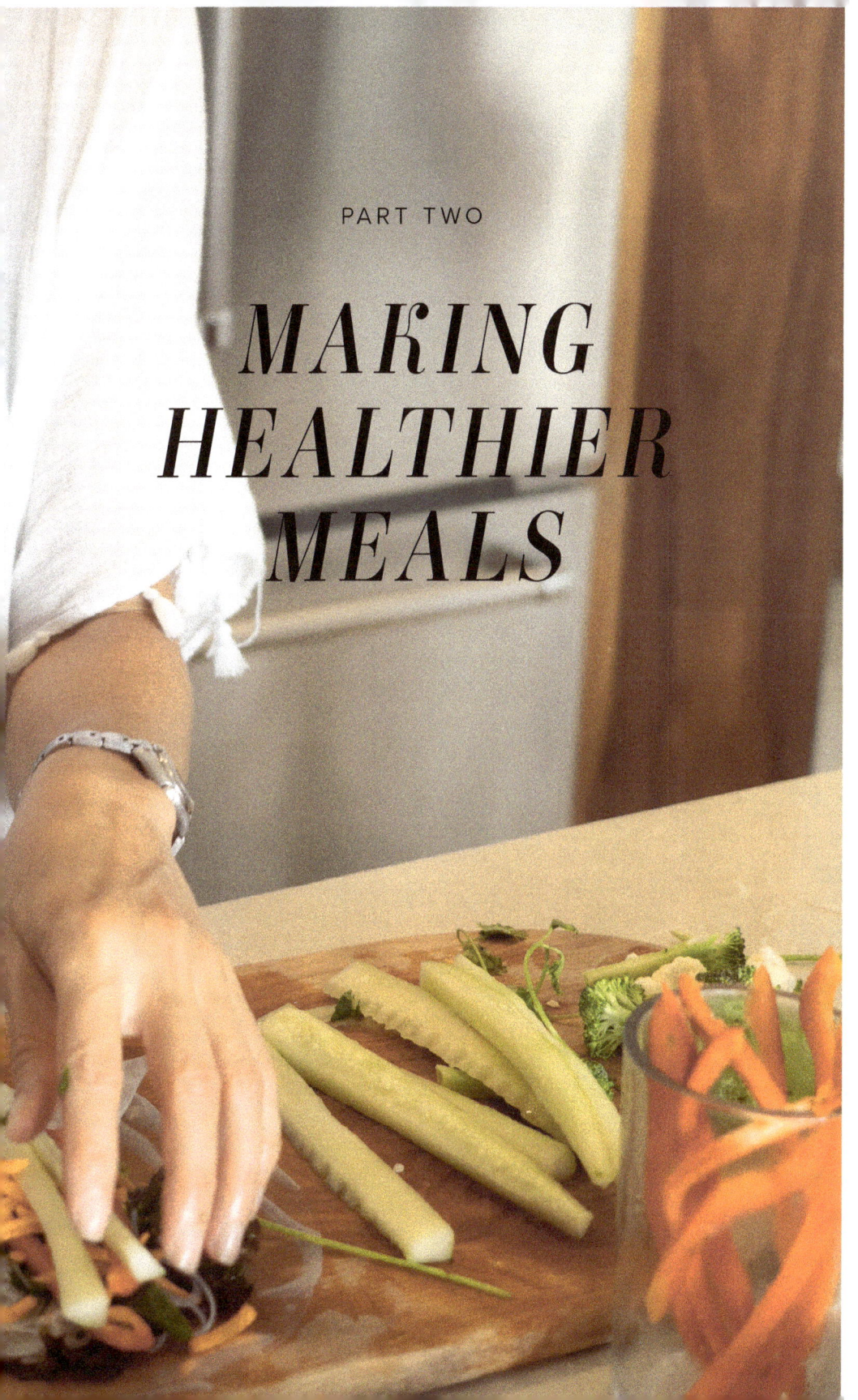

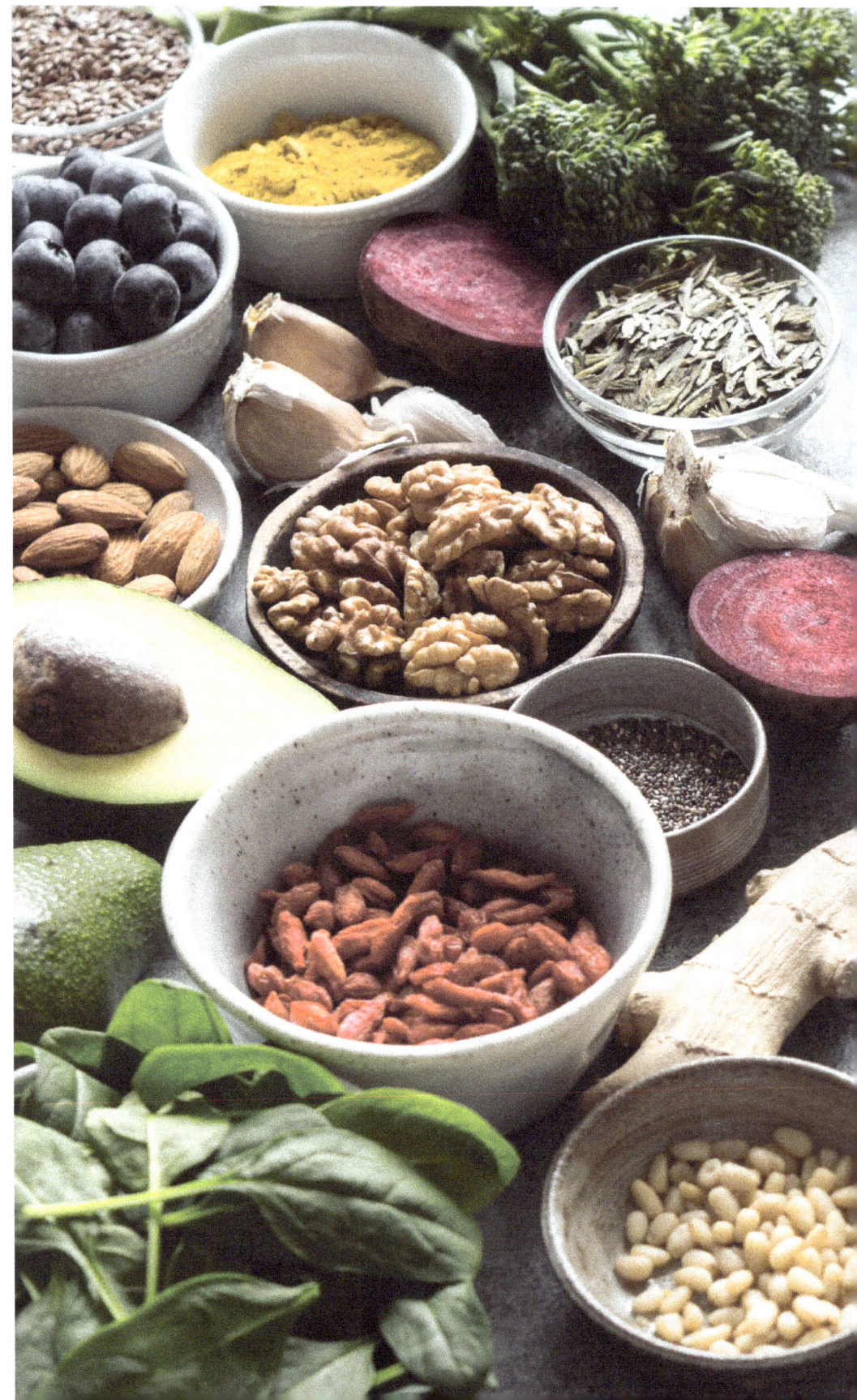

Anti-Inflammatory
Recipes to Help You Feel Better,
Be Stronger, and Live longer

An anti-inflammatory diet is one of the most delicious, incorporating the rich flavors of the Mediterranean and beyond. The next time you're in the kitchen, whip up some of these simple, affordable, and seasonal recipes to help reduce inflammation for overall good health.

In a nutshell, anti-inflammatory foods include lots of fruits and vegetables, whole grains, plant-based proteins, fatty fish, nuts, seeds, and fresh herbs and spices. Go for a variety of organic, local produce loaded with lots of green, orange, and red colors. Leafy greens like spinach and kale curb inflammation, as does broccoli. The substance that gives red grapes, cherries, blueberries, and raspberries their color is a type of pigment that also helps fight inflammation. Organically grown foods are nutrient-dense foods, which perform better under extreme weather conditions such as drought and floods. Better for the environment too!

These gluten-free recipes are mostly vegan, with a few fish options. They are simple, tasty, and healthy. You can make extra soup and stew which can be refrigerated or frozen for future use. Feel free to substitute ingredients in certain recipes, like adding spinach instead of kale, or cashew milk if you're out of almond. The idea is to be creative and have fun in the kitchen.

Let's get cooking!

Juice & Smoothies

GREEN JUICE

VEGAN

2   green apples
3   kale or Swiss chard leaves
1 fennel bulb
½ cucumber
1 cup parsley leaves
1 peeled lemon
1 teaspoon spirulina (optional)

Wash vegetables and fruit and chop into pieces small enough to fit easily down the chute of your juicer. I recommend peeling all citrus fruits. Turn your machine on and run all ingredients through the juicer, using your tamper as needed.

Tip: If you don't have fresh kale, you can substitute frozen or use other leafy greens such as spinach.

CARROT AND BEET CLEANSING JUICE

VEGAN

2 beets
½ daikon
4 carrots, medium to large
4 apples, cored and sliced
2.5 cm (1 in) fresh ginger
2.5 cm (1 in) turmeric root, peeled and sliced

Wash vegetables and fruit and chop into pieces small enough to fit easily down the chute of your juicer. Turn your machine on and run all ingredients through the juicer, using your tamper as needed.

Tip: If you can't find fresh turmeric, you could use 1 teaspoon of turmeric powder.

TURMERIC AND GINGER SMOOTHIE

VEGAN

½ cup fresh or frozen mango
1 banana, preferably frozen
1 teaspoon grated ginger
1 teaspoon grated turmeric
1 scoop vegan protein or colla-
    gen powder (optional)

In a blender, combine all ingredients with 1 cup of filtered
water or nut milk and blend.

Tip: feel free to substitute fresh or
frozen pineapple for the mango.
I often use organic oat milk for
this recipe.

SUNRISE SMOOTHIE

VEGAN

1 cup baby kale or spinach
½ avocado
1 cup pineapple
1 scoop vegan protein or colla-
    gen powder (optional)

In a blender, combine all ingredients with 1 cup of filtered
water or non-dairy milk and
blend.

Tip: Add ½ teaspoon of spirulina
and a few hemp hearts for a little
extra nutrition.

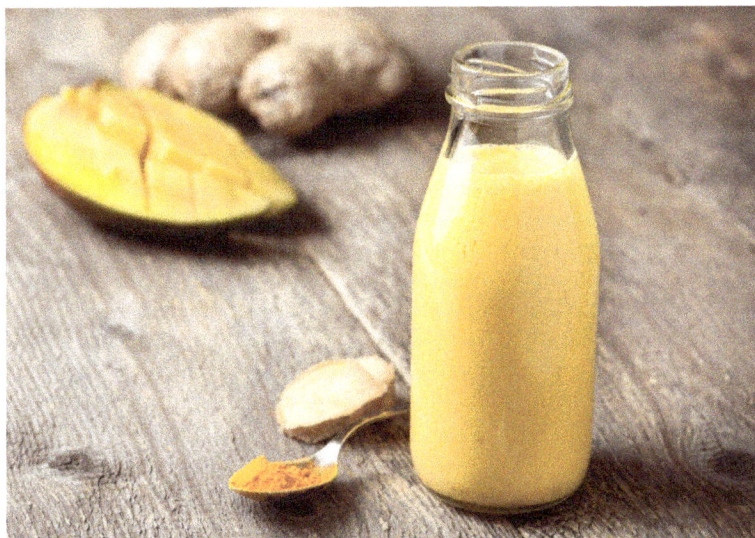

HOME-BREWED KOMBUCHA

VEGAN

13 cups filtered water
1 tablespoon loose-leaf black tea
1 tablespoon loose-leaf green tea
1 cup coconut sugar or 1 cup honey
1 cup starter kombucha from previous batch or store-bought
1 kombucha scoby

1   Bring 4 cups of filtered water to boil. Pour into a jar. Use a tea strainer to steep the leaves in the boiling water for about ten minutes. Add the sugar or honey, stir well and add the remaining 9 cups of filtered water.

2   Add the starter kombucha and the scoby. Stretch a piece of cloth over the opening of the jar and secure with a rubber band. Keep the jar in a dark place to ferment for 7–10 days. The hotter it is, the quicker it will ferment. You can start testing it after a week.

3   Split into smaller jars or bottles and add your favorite flavors.

Tip: I love using fresh ginger, citrus juice, or mint to flavor my homemade kombucha.

Breakfast

CHIA PUDDING

VEGAN

1 cup oat or nut milk of your choice
2 tablespoons chia seeds
1 tablespoon honey or maple syrup (optional)

Start with two small mason jars of milk and mix chia seeds and sweetener very well. You may prefer to sweeten it only with fruit, nuts, or dark chocolate. Place in the fridge for at least 2 hours to up to 6 days. If the chia pudding is too thick, you can add a little extra nut milk or coconut kefir.

Tip: I sometimes add a tablespoon of granola to the milk mixture.

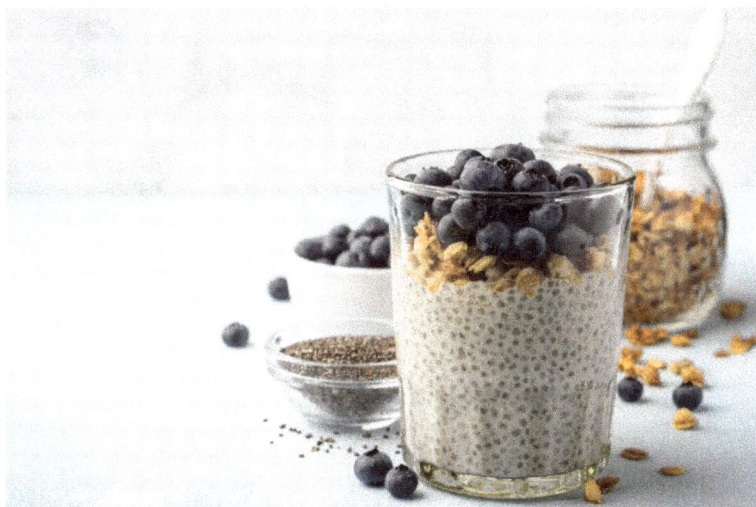

QUINOA GRANOLA

VEGAN

2 cups gluten-free, rolled oats
1 cup quinoa flakes — if quinoa flakes are not easy to find,
    simply use additional oats
⅓ cup shredded coconut
1 tablespoon hemp hearts
1 tablespoon chia seeds
¼ cup sesame seeds
⅓ cup slivered almonds
⅓ cup chopped walnuts, pecans, or hazelnuts
2 tablespoons coconut butter
4 tablespoons unpasteurized honey or maple syrup
½ tablespoon cinnamon
Pinch of sea salt
½ cup dark chocolate chunks or dried fruit of your choice

1 Preheat oven to 180 °C (350 °f).
2 Prepare two large baking sheets by lining them with parchment paper.
3 In a saucepan, over medium heat, combine honey or maple syrup and coconut butter until the mixture is melted.
4 In a large bowl, combine the rest of the ingredients. Set dried fruit aside for once the granola has cooled.
5 Pour the honey mixture over the top and mix.
6 Spread the granola evenly over the two baking sheets and place in the hot oven. Bake for about twenty to thirty minutes, stirring occasionally.
7 Let cool and add the dark chocolate or dried fruit, such as cherries, blueberries, or cranberries.

Tip: Be creative and have fun with this recipe. Substitute any nuts, seeds, and dried fruit you can find in your pantry. Can be served with milk, yogurt, or ice cream.

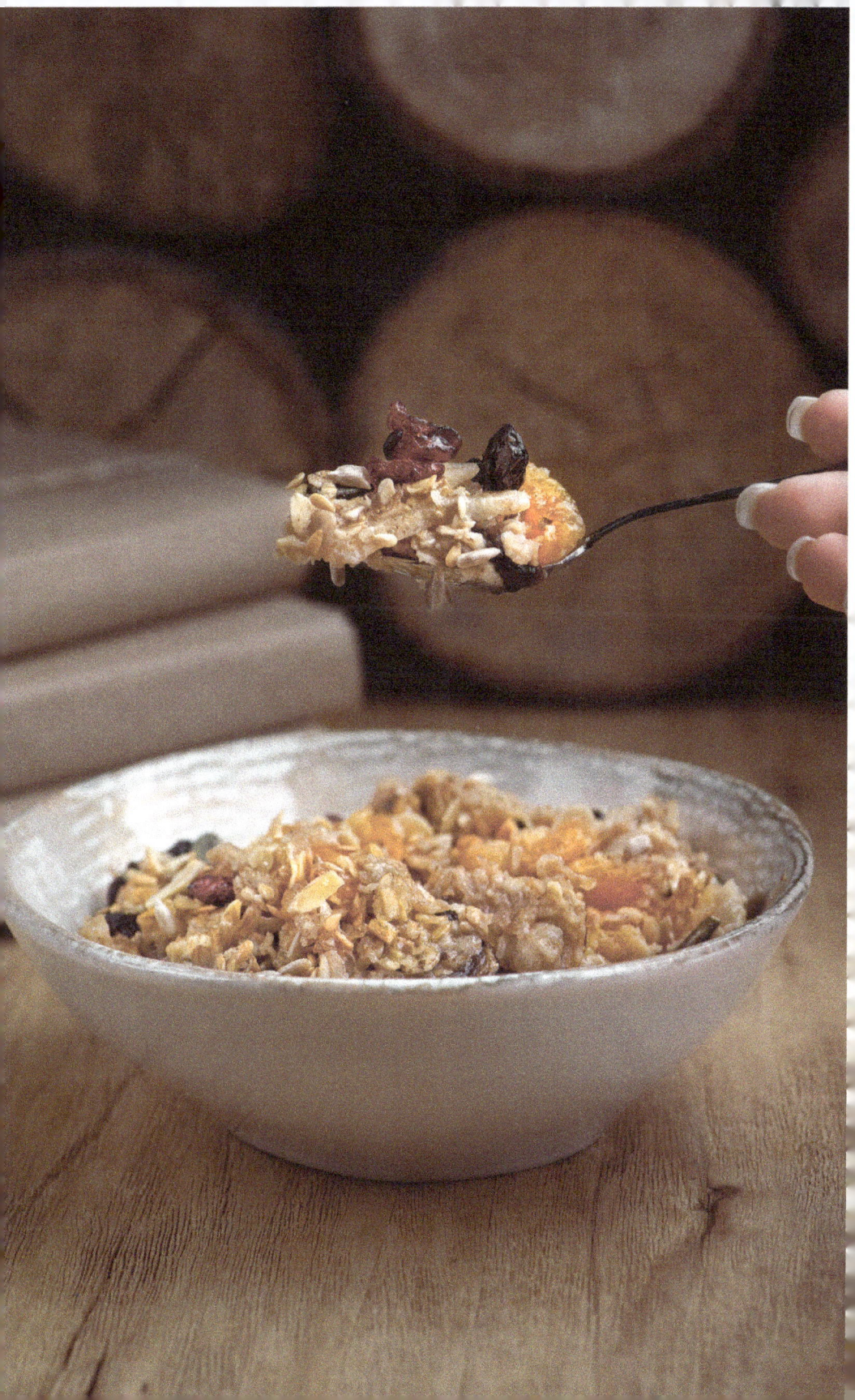

NUTTY BREAKFAST PORRIDGE

VEGAN

¾ cup gluten-free, rolled oats
1½ cups water or non-dairy milk
¼ teaspoon ground cinnamon
2 tablespoons chopped nuts, such as
    walnuts, pecans, or cashews
2 tablespoons dried fruit, such as
    raisins, cranberries, chopped apples
Maple syrup or honey (optional)
Pinch sea salt

1   Combine the oats and 1½ cups water in a small saucepan. Add
    chopped apples and cranberries or raisins. Bring to a boil over
    high heat. Reduce the heat to medium-low and cook until the
    water has been absorbed; this should take about fifteen minutes.
2   Stir in the cinnamon and salt. Top with nuts or seeds of your
    choice. If desired, pour a little maple syrup on top or add a little
    nut milk.

Tip: You can skip the fruit in the cooking process and add fresh berries or
sliced banana as a topper at the end.

Dips & Hummus

WHITE BEAN AND TRUFFLE OIL DIP

VEGAN

¼ cup olive oil
1 tablespoon truffle oil, plus additional for topping
3 large garlic cloves, diced
1 tablespoon parsley, finely chopped
2 cans cannellini beans, drained and rinsed
3 tablespoons fresh lemon juice
Salt and pepper to taste
Optional toppings: pine nuts, fresh thyme, red pepper flakes

1   Heat olive oil in a pan over medium heat. Add garlic and sauté for
    two to three minutes.
2   Add beans, olive oil and parsley, lemon juice, and salt and pepper
    to a food processor.
3   Blend on high until dip is smooth and creamy.
4   Taste and adjust seasonings as needed, adding more salt, lemon
    juice, or olive oil if needed. If it's too thick, add a bit of water.
5   Drizzle truffle oil on top.

Tip: You can substitute the truffle oil for olive oil or add roasted garlic or
caramelized onion to mix it up sometimes.

GUACAMOLE

VEGAN

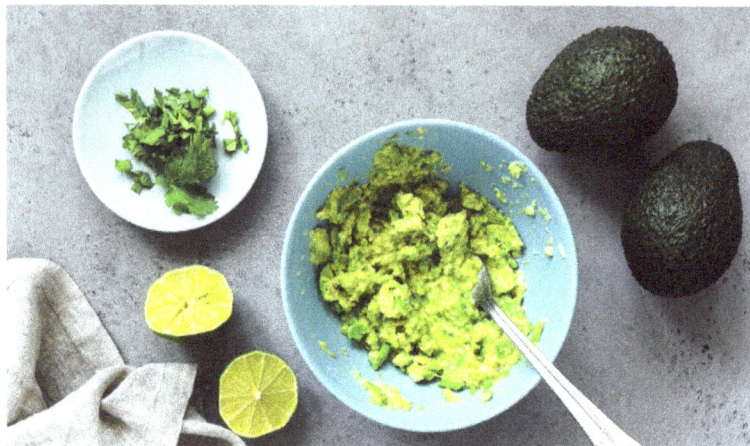

3 avocados
2 tablespoons fresh lime juice
¼ small red onion, finely chopped
¼ cup cilantro, finely chopped
Sea salt and black pepper to taste

1   Slice the avocados in half and remove the core. Scoop out the flesh into a bowl and then mash with a fork.
2   Add the fresh lime juice and mash.
3   Add the chopped red onion, diced cherry tomatoes, and chopped cilantro and mix in.
4   Add sea salt and black pepper to taste. Add hot sauce if you want to spice it up a bit.
5   Serve with tortilla chips or sliced raw vegetables.

. . . .

Tip: If you put the avocado pit in the guacamole, it keeps the dip from going brown as fast.

BEET HUMMUS

VEGAN

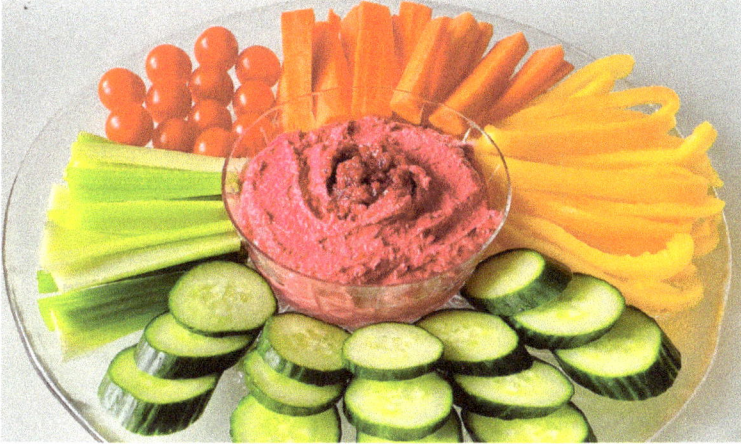

2 roasted or boiled beets
1 400 g (15 oz) can chickpeas, drained
1 large lemon, juiced and zested
2 large cloves garlic, minced
2 tablespoons tahini
¼ cup extra virgin olive oil
Salt and pepper to taste

1 Once your beets are cooled and peeled, place them in your food processer. Blend until only small bits remain.
2 Add remaining ingredients except olive oil and blend until smooth.
3 Drizzle in olive oil as the hummus is mixing.
4 Taste and adjust seasonings as needed, adding more salt, lemon juice or olive oil if needed. If it's too thick, add a bit of water.

Tip: It usually keeps well in the refrigerator for a week, so I usually double up on the recipe. I also substitute the beets for caramelized onions or roasted garlic sometimes.

Soups & Stews

CURRIED PUMPKIN SOUP

VEGAN

2 tablespoons red curry paste
4 cups vegetable broth
2 400 g (15 oz) cans pumpkin puree (or make your own)
1¾ cups coconut milk
Roasted pumpkin seeds as garnish if desired

1   In a Dutch oven or large saucepan, cook the curry paste over medium heat for about one minute or until paste becomes fragrant. Add 2 cups of broth and the pumpkin and stir.
2   I made this soup the other day using a fresh kabocha pumpkin, which is green on the outside and orange on the inside. Slice the pumpkin in half, scoop out the seeds, and drizzle with olive oil. Place on a baking sheet and bake at 190 °C (375 °f) for about fifty minutes or until the flesh is soft. Let cool and scoop out into the food processor with a cup of broth and puree.
3   Add the pumpkin mix to the pan with the curry paste. Add the coconut milk and cook until hot (about three minutes). Partway through cooking, check the liquid levels and, if you need to, add the remaining broth or a little bit of water.
4   Ladle into bowls and garnish with a drizzle of the coconut milk and roasted pumpkin seeds if desired.

Tip: My kids love this soup! worth doubling the recipe and freezing it.

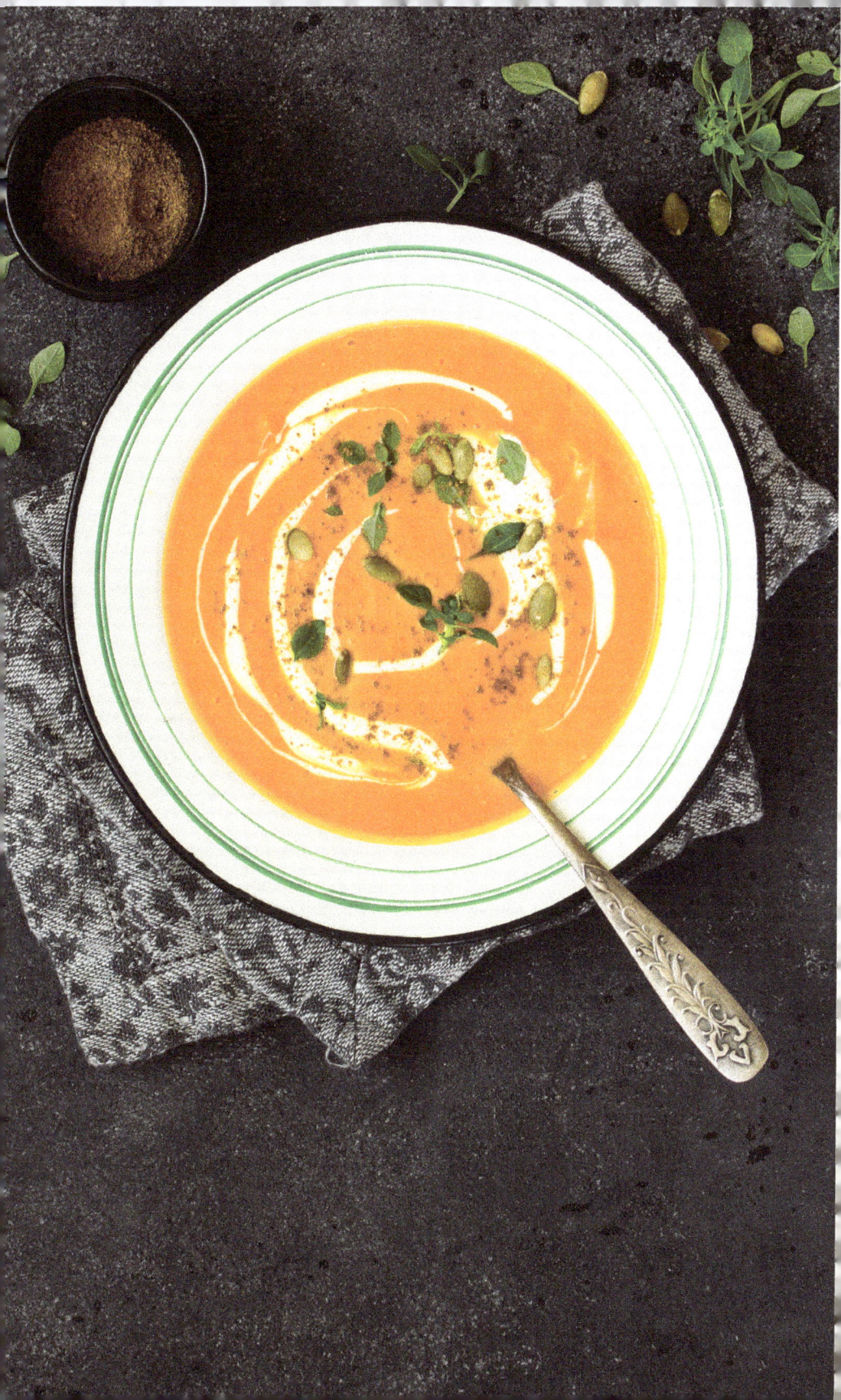

LOUISE'S MISO MUSHROOM SOUP

VEGAN

3 packages mushrooms, one each of: shiitake,
  portobello, brown, or any other mushroom
1 onion, chopped
3 garlic cloves, minced
1 teaspoon dry garlic powder
Olive oil
¼ cup **Madeira wine**
1 cup white wine
2 cubes concentrated mushroom soup
1 tablespoon miso
6 cups vegetable broth
¼ cup minced parsley

1   Heat the oil in a soup pot, and add the onion and garlic. Cook until
    lightly browned. Add the cut-up mushrooms and brown lightly on
    medium to high heat, turning as little as possible to keep them
    browning.

2   Add the Madeira and the white wine, the cubed mushroom soup
    concentrate, the vegetable broth, the garlic powder, and the miso.
    Bring to a simmer and let cook on low for approximately thirty
    to forty minutes. Adjust seasoning and add pepper. Turn off heat.
    Take 2 cups of the soup and pulse in a blender. Serve with the
    parsley as garnish.

GINGER AND CARROT SOUP

VEGAN

2 tablespoons olive oil
1 leek, cleaned and chopped
1 parsnip, peeled and chopped
3 cups chopped carrots
1 cup chopped butternut squash (or other squash)
2 garlic cloves, minced
2 tablespoons grated ginger
1 teaspoon turmeric powder
3-4 cups low-sodium vegetable broth,
depending on desired thickness
1 cup unsweetened coconut milk
Salt and pepper to taste

1   Heat the olive oil in a large Dutch oven or saucepan. Add the leeks, carrots, and squash. Sauté for three to five minutes until the veggies start to soften. Add the garlic, ginger, turmeric, salt, and pepper, and sauté for a few more minutes.

2   Add the broth and coconut milk. Bring the mixture to a boil, cover, and simmer for twenty minutes. Partway through cooking, check the liquid levels and, if you need to, add a little bit of hot water.

3   Once the soup is cooked, add it to a blender and blend until creamy. You could also use an immersion blender. Taste and adjust seasonings to your taste.

Tip: If you are not a fan of coconut milk, simply add extra broth. I've made this soup using sweet potatoes instead of squash.

KALE AND WHITE BEAN STEW

VEGAN

500g (1 lb) dried cannellini beans, soaked and drained
6 cups vegetable broth
1 cup chopped yellow onion
2 garlic cloves, chopped
1 cup sliced carrots
1 teaspoon finely chopped rosemary
4 cups chopped kale
1 tablespoon fresh lemon juice
3 tablespoons extra virgin olive oil
¼ cup parsley leaves
Parmesan, grated, and 7 cm (3 in) piece rind (optional)
Salt and pepper to taste

1 Fry onions, garlic, and carrots in the olive oil for five minutes on medium.
2 Add broth, beans, rosemary, and parmesan rind. Cover and cook on low for about 1 hour.
3 Stir in kale. Cover and cook on high until the kale is tender.
4 Stir in lemon juice, salt, and pepper. Discard the parmesan rind. Serve the stew with fresh parmesan and parsley.

Tip: worth doubling the recipe and freezing.

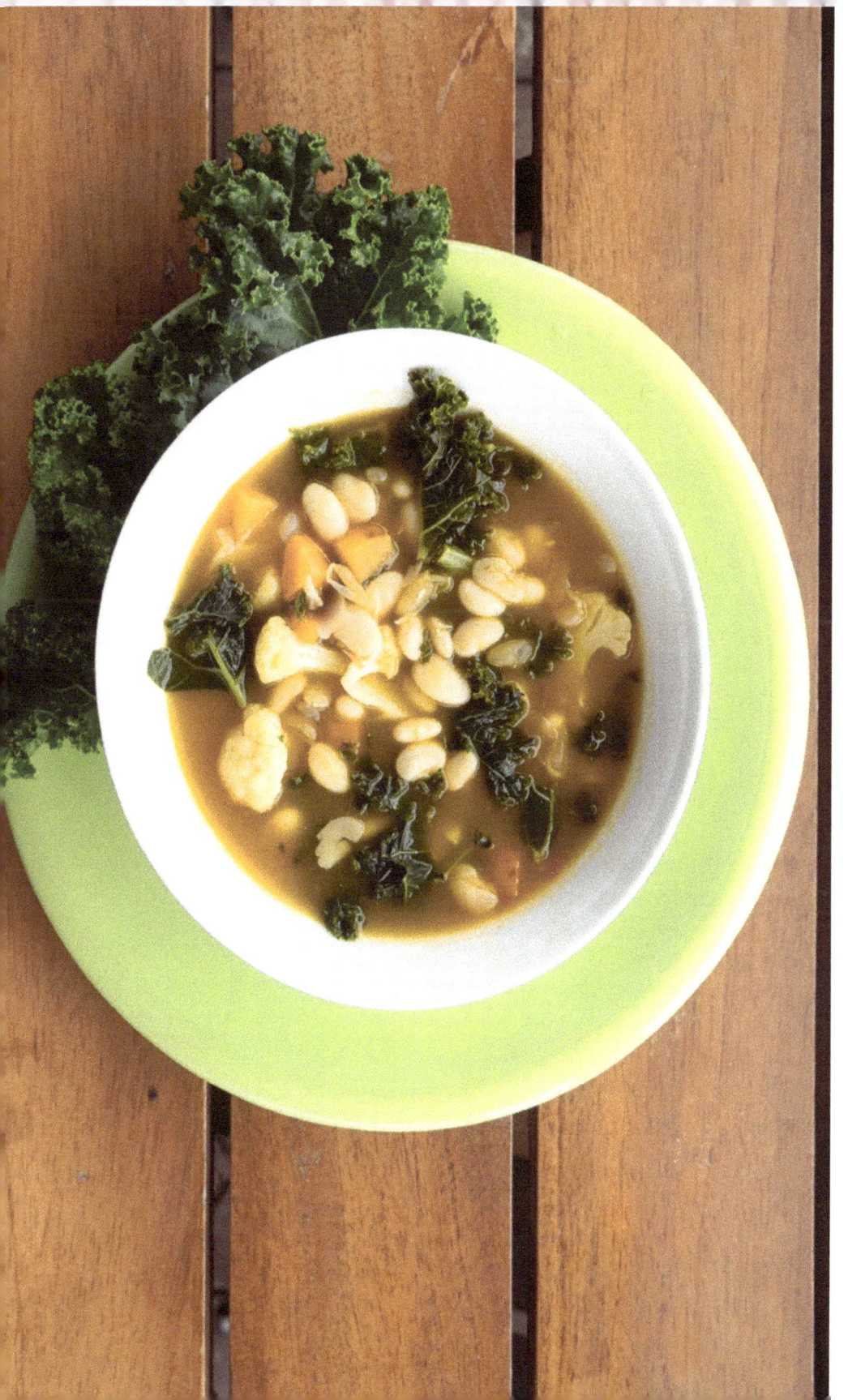

Salsa & Salads

MANGO SALSA

VEGAN

3 mangos, peeled and thinly sliced
1 red bell pepper, thinly sliced
¼ red onion, thinly sliced
¼ cup fresh cilantro, roughly chopped

DRESSING
⅓ cup fresh lime juice (about 3 limes)
⅛ teaspoon red pepper flakes
2 tablespoons sesame oil
Salt and pepper to taste
½ cup cashews (topping)

1   Combine all the ingredients for the mango salsa in a large bowl. Toss to combine.
2   Prepare the dressing by combining all the ingredients in a small bowl and whisking well. Cover and refrigerate if making ahead or use immediately by drizzling over the salad and tossing to combine. Add cashews at the very end.

Tip: I sometimes omit the cashews in this recipe and chop the mangos up into chunks or substitute them for pineapple. Accompanies fish well!

CHICKPEA SALAD

VEGAN

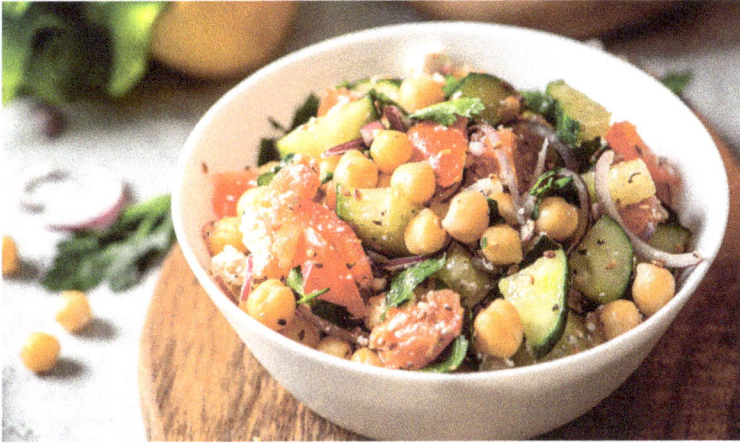

1 small red onion, peeled and chopped

2 celery sticks, peeled and chopped

10 cherry tomatoes

1 red bell pepper, seeded and chopped

1 English cucumber, peeled and chopped

1 can of chickpeas

2 tablespoons extra virgin olive oil

2 lemons, juiced

2 cloves pressed garlic

1 teaspoon dried basil

1 teaspoon dried oregano

Sea salt and pepper to taste

Place all the ingredients in a salad bowl and toss.

Tip: My vegetarian daughter loves chickpea salad. I'm always mixing it up by adding feta and/or quinoa. If you're sensitive to nightshades, you'll want to omit the tomatoes and peppers.

BEET AND WALNUT SALAD

2 medium beets, cooked, peeled, and diced
⅓ cup toasted walnuts
1 275 g (10 oz) package mixed greens
½ red onion, thinly sliced
⅓ cup extra virgin olive oil
¼ cup balsamic vinegar
¼ cup pomegranate seeds or dried cranberries
Crumbled goat's cheese, if desired
Pinch of sea salt and pepper

1   Place beets in the oven at 180 °C (350 °f) or in a saucepan with enough water to cover and bring to boil. Cook for twenty to thirty minutes or until tender. Roasting in the oven will take slightly longer but they will have a bit more flavor. Cool the beets, dice, and set aside.

2   In a small bowl, whisk balsamic vinegar and olive oil to make the dressing. Season to taste with sea salt and black pepper.

3   Place all the ingredients in a salad bowl and toss.

Tip: Mix it up by using toasted pumpkin seeds or pecans. Try cooking extra beets and refrigerating for future use.

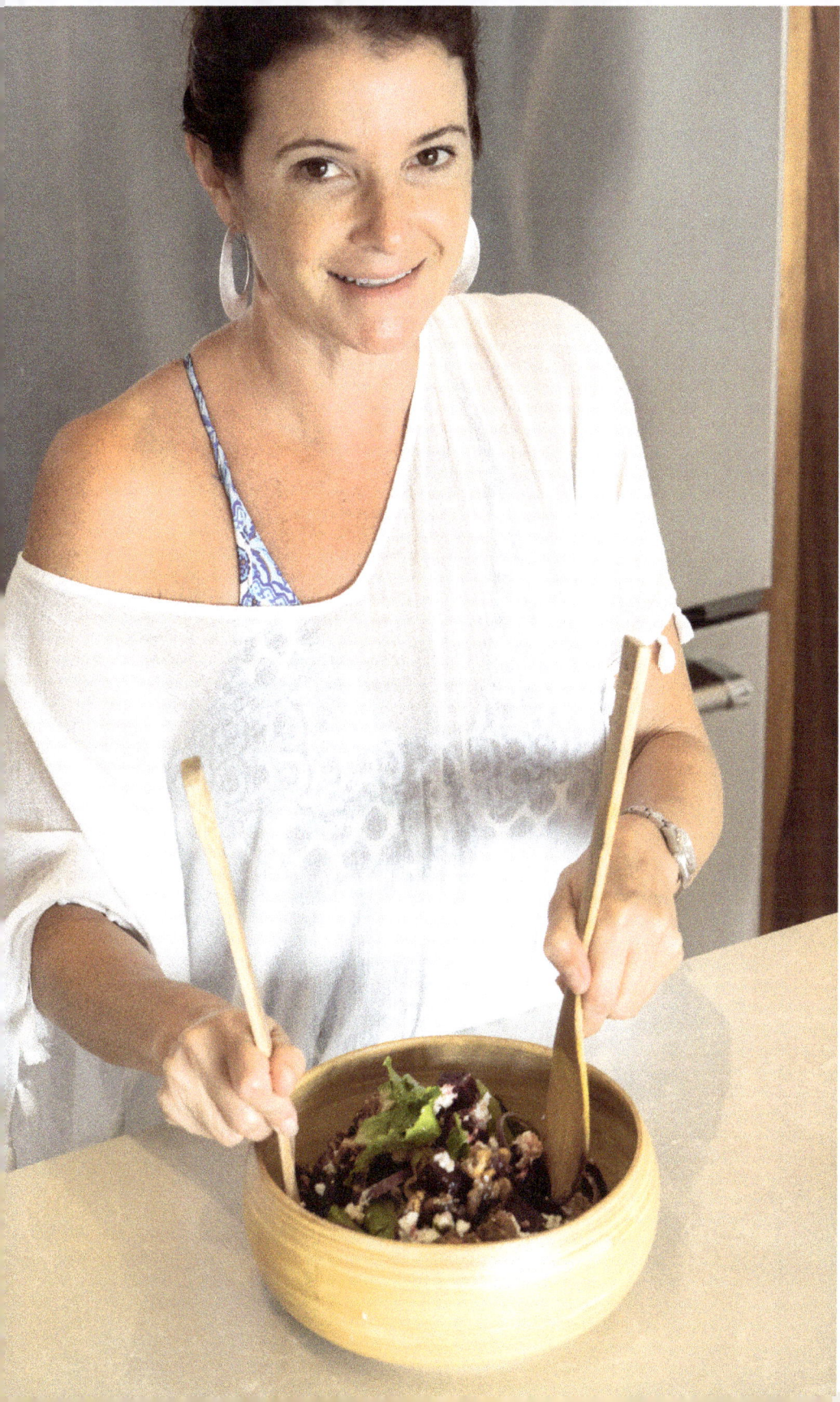

Buddha Bowl, Rice & Rolls

BUDDHA BOWL

VEGAN

1¼ cups brown rice or quinoa
2 limes, juiced
2 tablespoons sesame oil
1 cup frozen, shelled edamame, preferably organic
1½ cups trimmed and roughly chopped snap peas or snow peas,
    or thinly sliced broccoli
1 cup chopped red cabbage or macrobiotic slaw (from page 108)
1 cup leafy greens
1 ripe avocado, halved, pitted and thinly sliced
1 small cucumber, very thinly sliced
Salt and pepper to taste
¼ cup pesto (see recipe below) to flavor the quinoa

1   Add the pesto, edamame, and peas or broccoli to the cooked
    brown rice or quinoa.
2   Divide the rice/veggie mixture and raw veggies into four bowls.
    Arrange cucumber slices along the edge of the bowl. Drizzle lightly
    with olive oil and lime juice.
3   When you're ready to serve, divide the avocado into the bowls.
    Season with salt and pepper.

Tip: Try substituting the quinoa for brown rice occasionally. Omit the pesto
if you wish and simply season with extra vinaigrette. Feel free to add other
veggies you have kicking around.

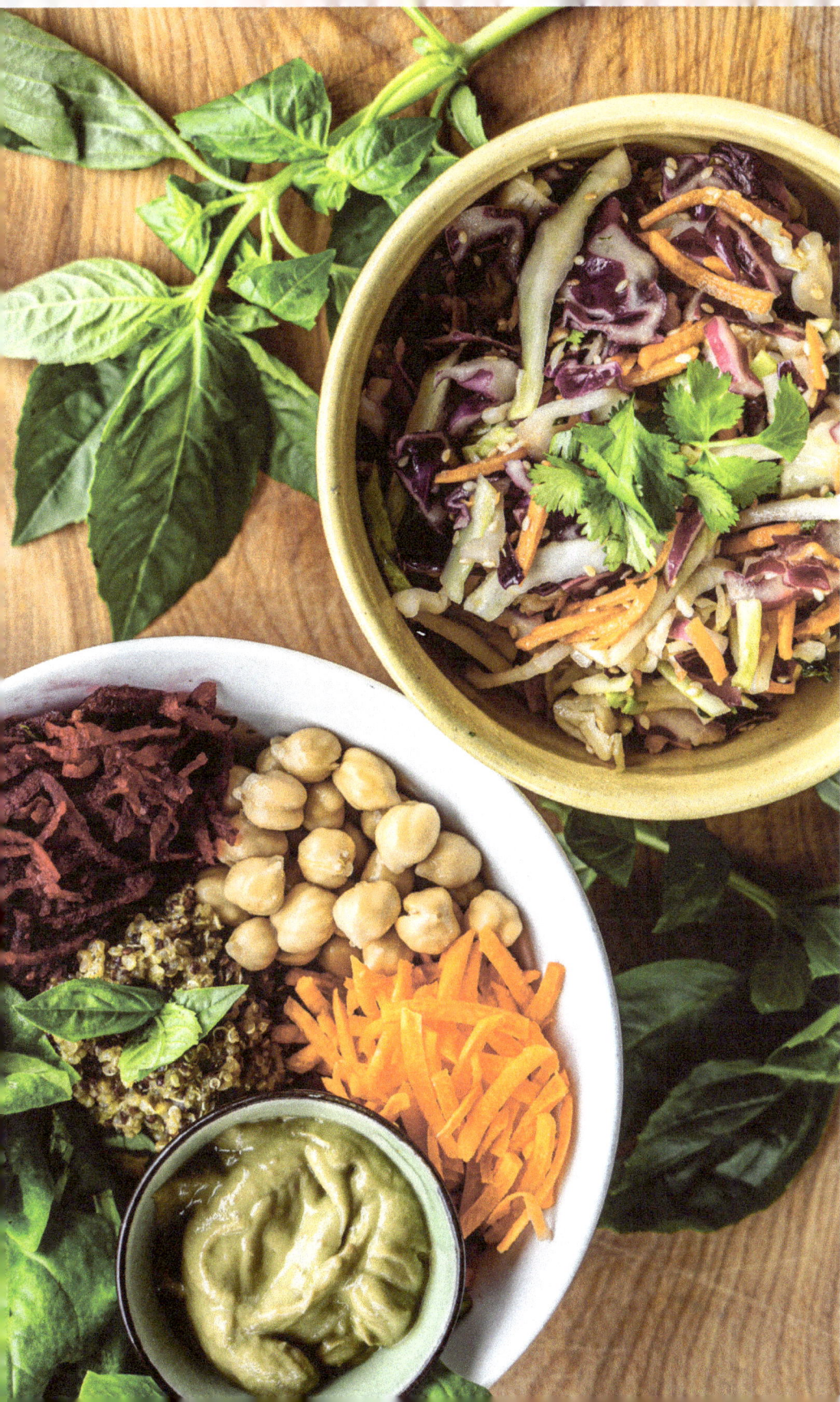

PESTO

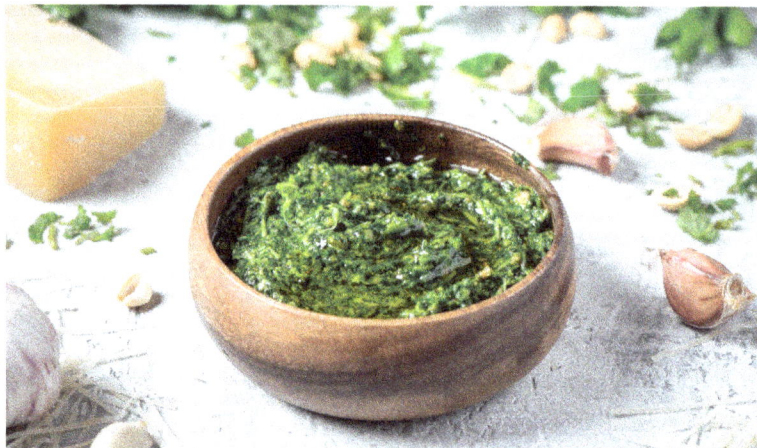

1 cup fresh basil or parsley leaves
3 cloves garlic, peeled
3 tablespoons pine nuts
⅓ cup freshly grated parmesan or vegan hard cheese
Salt and freshly ground black pepper, to taste
⅓ cup olive oil

Combine basil or parsley, garlic, nuts, and parmesan in the bowl of a food processor; season with salt and pepper to taste. With the motor running, add olive oil until it is emulsified.

Tip: Store pesto in an airtight container in the refrigerator for up to one week, or freeze. My kids love this pesto when I serve it with big egg noodles, toasted pine nuts, and broccoli.

RICE PILAF WITH NUTS

VEGAN

2 tablespoons avocado or olive oil
Pinch sea salt and pepper to season
2 celery sticks, chopped
1 onion, peeled and chopped
1 clove garlic, finely chopped
1 carrot, peeled and chopped
1 cup basmati rice or brown rice
2 cups vegetable stock
¾ cup unsalted nuts (cashews or almonds)
Parsley or cilantro (optional garnish)

1   In a large frying pan, on medium heat, combine onions, garlic, celery, and carrots in the olive oil until they are soft.
2   Add the vegetable stock and bring to boil. Reduce heat to low, add the rice, and cover for about thirty to forty minutes. Partway through cooking, check the liquid levels and, if you need to, add a little bit of hot water.
3   Once cooked, let sit for about five minutes and add the nuts, salt, pepper, and some parsley or cilantro as a garnish.

Tip: Try substituting the rice with quinoa. You can also use leftover rice by simply adding it to the cooked veggies with a little bit of broth.

RICE PAPER ROLLS

VEGAN

8 rice paper wrappers
1 medium cucumber
1 medium bell pepper
1 mango
2 medium carrots
Leafy greens
Fresh mint
Fresh cilantro

DIPPING SAUCE
3 tablespoons sesame oil
2 cloves garlic, peeled
2 tablespoons tamari
1–2 tablespoons all-natural peanut butter
1 tablespoon water
1 tablespoon honey
2 limes, juiced
Optional: Add shrimp or tofu if you wish

1 Place the ingredients for the peanut sauce in a food processor or blender and blend until smooth.
2 If you have an issue with peanuts, you could try hoisin sauce as a dipping sauce.
3 Julienne or slice the mango, cucumber, pepper, and carrots into thin strips. A mandolin slicer is perfect.
4 Soak one rice paper wrapper at a time in a bowl of warm water for a few seconds. When you see or feel the wrapper getting loose, remove it from the water and set it on a plate.
5 Arrange a few leafy greens on the rice paper and add the vegetables and herbs in the center of the wrapper. Fold the sides towards the middle, fold the top flap over the vegetables, and roll.

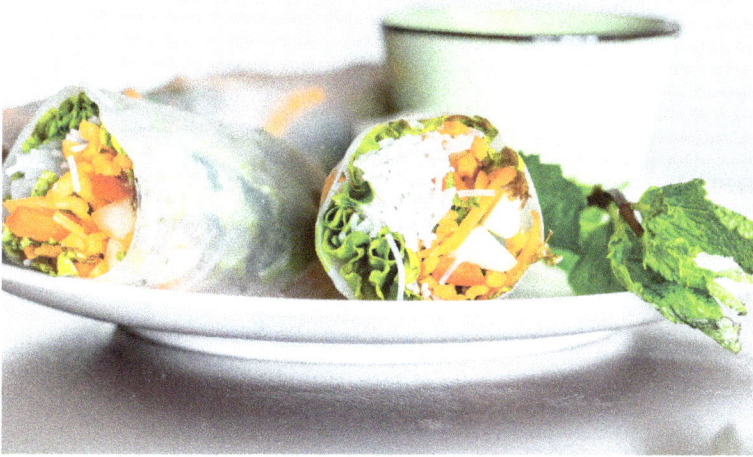
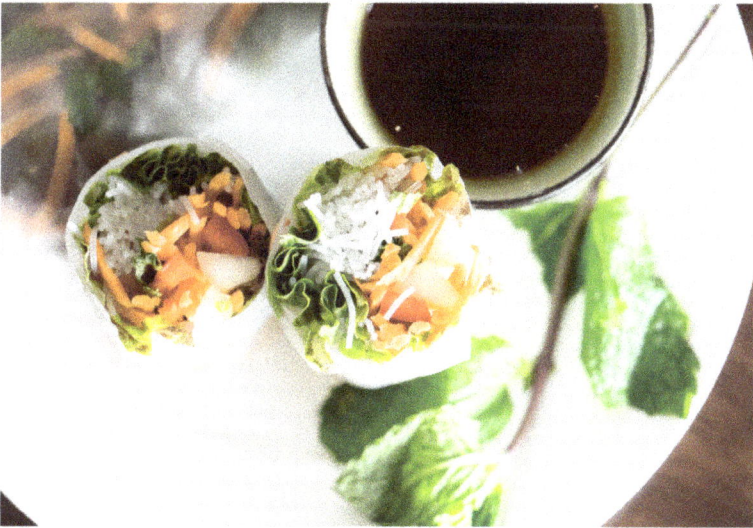

Tip: Add tofu, cashews or shrimp in the wraps. I sometime exclude the rice paper and turn them into lettuce wraps for a change.

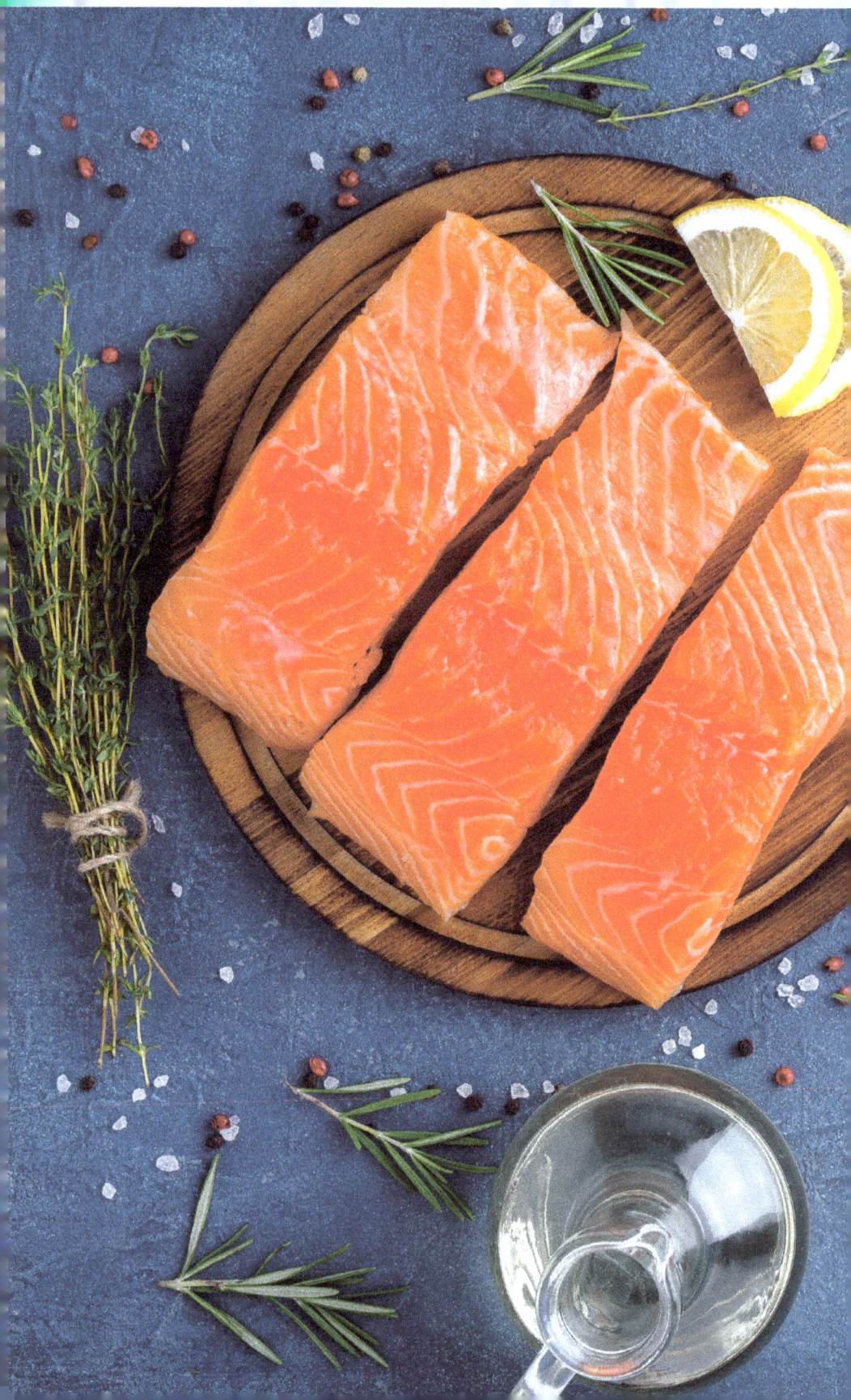

Wild Sustainable Seafood

Fish supplies a large amount of the omega-3 fatty acids that have been shown to cut the risk of heart attack and stroke. Omega-3s may also elevate mood and help prevent certain cancers, cognitive decline, and eye disease. Most people can get enough by consuming fatty fish at least twice a week. Good choices include wild salmon, trout, and sardines since they're also low in mercury. Mercury-containing plants and tiny animals are eaten by smaller fish that are then gobbled up by larger fish, whose tissue accumulates the toxin.

The larger, longer-living predators such as sharks and swordfish tend to have more of the toxin than smaller fish. Large amounts of mercury can harm the nervous system of a fetus or young child. While the health effects of sporadic exposure are unclear, fish safety experts think that women who are pregnant or nursing, as well as young children, should take special precautions when it comes to what fish they eat.

The fish and shellfish in supermarkets are harvested in ways that are ecologically disastrous. Bottom trawling scrapes the seafloor clean. According to the World Wildlife Federation, the number of fish in the ocean has fallen by half since 1970, and ninety percent of the world's fisheries are overexploited.

Is it possible to enjoy your seafood without the toxins and mercury? Go to one of the many websites like https://seafood.ocean.org/seafood/ or www.fda.gov/food/consumers/advice-about-eating-fish for recommendations.

Seafood

MARINATED SALMON WITH SLAW

4 fish fillets
2 limes, juiced, plus 1 lime for garnish
2 tablespoons olive oil, plus 1 tablespoon for marinade
Sea salt and pepper

1   Combine the fish, lime juice, oil and salt, and pepper in a bowl and let marinate for six hours.
2   Heat a large cast-iron skillet over medium-high heat. Add olive oil, then, when hot, add the fish. Carefully flip with a thin, wide spatula and cook on the other side until the fish is golden brown, nearly opaque, and flakes easily with a fork.
3   Serve with lime wedges, for squeezing over the top of the pan-fried salmon.

Tip: Try trout instead of salmon.

MACROBIOTIC SLAW
2 cups thinly sliced Asian cabbage
1 cup thinly sliced red cabbage
1 cup thinly sliced bok choy
3 scallions, sliced
½ cup cilantro, chopped
¼ cup toasted sesame seeds or cashews

MISO DRESSING

2 tablespoons sesame oil

1 tablespoon white miso

2 tablespoons non-dairy milk (cashew or oat)

¼ cup rice wine vinegar or lime juice

1 garlic clove, minced

Salt and pepper to taste

1 Toss slaw ingredients together in a large bowl. Add cilantro and scallions.
2 Add dressing ingredients to a food processor and blend. Pour dressing into slaw and toss well.
3 Garnish with seeds and/or nuts.

Tip: I often have this detox salad for dinner with miso soup when I need a dietary reset.

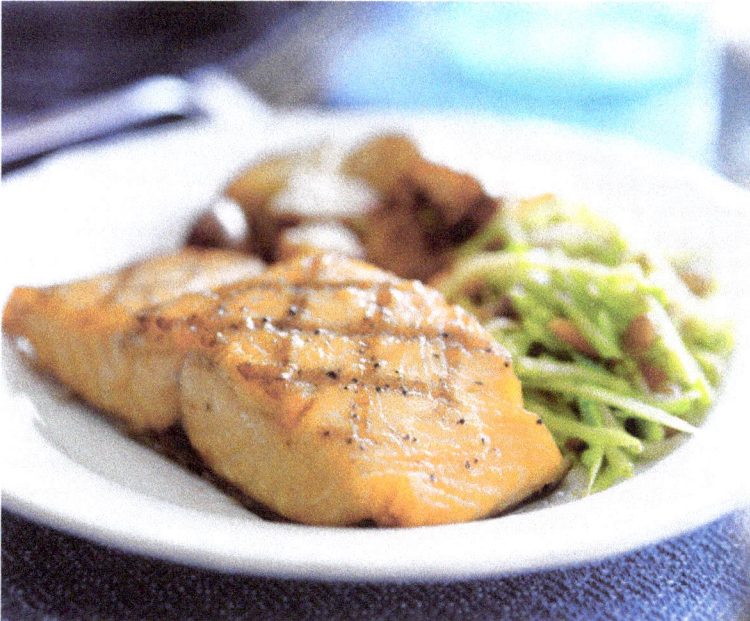

MISO COD WITH SPINACH AND MUSHROOMS

4 cod fillets about 3 cm (1.5 in) thick
2 tablespoons extra virgin olive oil
1 red onion
3 cloves garlic, minced
2 cups shiitake or mushrooms of your choice
275 g (10 oz) baby spinach
Salt and black pepper

MISO MARINADE

¼ cup sake
¼ mirin
3 tablespoon miso
2 tablespoons honey

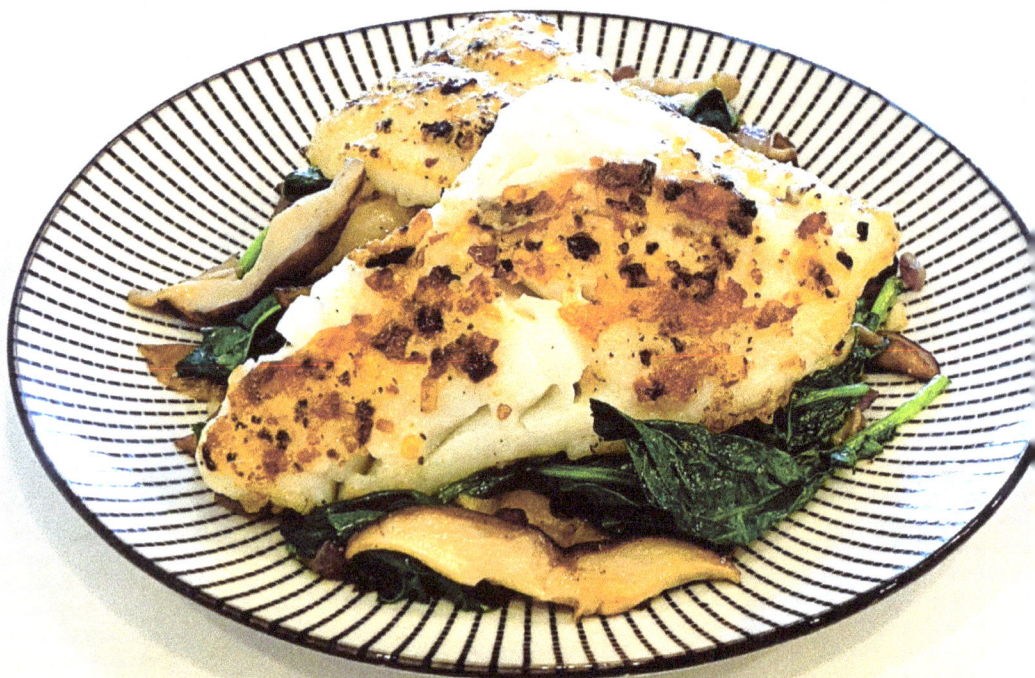

1 Boil sake and mirin until it reduces by a third. Add the honey and the miso at the end

2 Turn heat down and cook for two to three minutes, stirring constantly to prevent burning.

3 Cool to room temperature.

4 Marinate cod fillets in the miso mixture for one day.

5 Gently wipe off excess marinade from the fillets and grill or broil until well browned.

6 Heat the oil in a medium sauté pan over medium-low heat. Add the garlic and onions. Cook until fragrant, for about two minutes (do not let the garlic brown).

7 Add the mushrooms. Increase the heat to medium-high and season the mushrooms with salt and pepper to taste. Cook, stirring occasionally, until the mushrooms are cooked through, about ten to twelve minutes.

8 Add the spinach, turn with tongs until wilted, and serve.

Tip: You can substitute any low-mercury and sustainable white fish.

CHUCK'S SEARED TROUT AND SICILIAN FENNEL SALAD

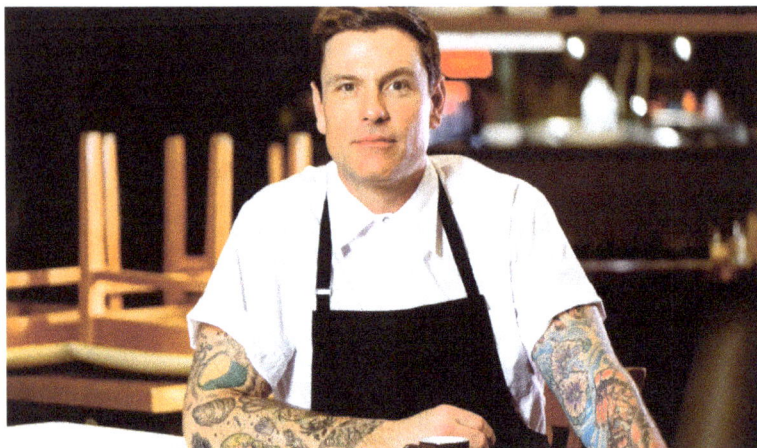

4 trout fillets
2 tablespoons olive oil
1 teaspoon fennel seeds, crushed
1 teaspoon dill seeds, crushed
1 teaspoon mustard seeds, crushed
1 teaspoon black pepper, crushed
Sea salt to taste
Lemon wedges, for serving

1 Pat the fish fillets dry with paper towels. Mix all the spices with a bit of olive oil and coat the top of the trout with this mixture.

2 Heat a large, cast-iron skillet over medium-high heat. Add the olive oil, then, when hot, lay the trout fillets spice-side down until crispy. Carefully flip with a thin, wide spatula and cook on the other side until the fish is golden brown, nearly opaque, and flakes easily with a fork.

3 Serve with lemon wedges, for squeezing over the top of the pan-fried trout.

Tip: Try this recipe with Arctic Char.

SICILIAN FENNEL SALAD

1 fennel bulb, very thinly sliced
2 celery sticks, very thinly sliced
2 large oranges
1 lemon, juiced
Parsley, finely chopped
3 tablespoons olive oil
Salt and pepper to taste

1   Cut the fennel in half and remove the core. Using a mandolin, thinly slice the fennel pieces. Place into a bowl.
2   Using a knife, thinly slice the celery at a diagonal and add to the bowl. Peel and cut one of the oranges and add the parsley to the bowl.
3   To make the dressing, you'll need to squeeze the juice out of the other orange and lemon. Combine citrus juice with olive oil. Season with salt and pepper.

Note: fennel is a good source of fiber, potassium, folate, vitamin C, vitamin B6, and phytonutrients. Fiber decreases the risk of heart disease as it helps reduce the total amount of cholesterol in the blood. The most fascinating phytonutrient compound in fennel, however, may be anethole—the primary component of its volatile oil. The volatile oil has also been shown to be able to protect the liver from toxic chemicals

FISH CAKES WITH TRUFFLE OIL

2 tablespoons olive oil
1 tablespoon truffle oil
100 g (3 ½ oz) boneless sustainable wild fish such as cod,
    salmon, trout
300 g (10 oz) sweet potatoes
A few sprigs fresh flat-leaf parsley
1 large free-range egg
1 lemon
Sea salt and pepper

1   Peel the potatoes, cut into chunks, and cook in boiling
    salted water for ten minutes.
2   Rub the fish with a little oil and a pinch of sea salt and black
    pepper and pan fry or bake in the oven. You can always use
    canned salmon if you want to skip this step.
3   Meanwhile, pick and finely chop the parsley leaves.
4   Once cooked, remove the fish from heat and discard the skin.
    Drain the potatoes and mash them.
5   Flake the fish into the bowl and add the egg, truffle oil,
    chopped parsley, and a pinch of sea salt and black pepper.
    Finely grate over the lemon zest, then mash and mix together
    really well.
6   Divide the mixture into four, then lightly shape and pat into circles
    about 2 cm (¾ in) thick. If you're going to freeze them, wrap them
    and put them into the freezer. Otherwise, pop them into the fridge
    for an hour before cooking to allow them to firm up slightly.
7   Heat oil in a large frying pan over medium heat, add the
    fishcakes, and cook five minutes on each side, or until crisp
    and golden.
8   Serve straight away, with lemon wedges for squeezing over.

Tip: Make extra and refrigerate or freeze for a later date.

ARCTIC CHAR WITH OVENROASTED VEGETABLES

2 tablespoons olive oil
2 tablespoons chopped mixed fresh herbs (such as parsley, thyme and rosemary)
Salt and pepper
1 cup sweet potatoes, cubed
2 parsnips, peeled and chopped
1 cup cauliflower florets
1 cup Brussels sprouts (about 10), trimmed and halved
700 g (1½ lb) Arctic Char fillet

1   Heat oven to 220 °C (425°f). In a bowl, whisk together oil, herbs, ¾ teaspoon salt, and ½ teaspoon pepper.

2   On a large rimmed baking sheet, toss potatoes, Brussels sprouts, and cauliflower with half of the oil mixture. Roast in the oven for twenty minutes before adding the Arctic Char fillet. Brush the fish with the remaining oil mixture and roast for a further fifteen to twenty minutes, until vegetables are golden brown and tender and Arctic Char is opaque throughout.

Tip: Try this recipe with wild salmon or trout. If you're lucky enough to find Jerusalem artichokes, also known as sunchokes, you can add them to the roasted root veggies. Parsnips and Jerusalem artichokes both provide a number of vitamins and minerals and may provide some health benefits because of their role as a prebiotic, promoting good gut bacteria.

Something Sweet

BAKED APPLE

VEGAN

4 medium-firm, cored apples
1 cup granola (make your own using the recipe on page 84)
¼ cup orange juice
Vanilla ice cream for serving

1 Preheat oven to 180 °C (350 °f). lightly spray a baking dish with non-stick spray or use parchment paper.
2 Take a knife and circle the apple horizontally, perforating the skin slightly. Scoop out the core, seeds, and stem. Arrange the apples in a baking dish. Mix the granola and juice. Fill the apples with the granola mixture.
3 Cover with aluminum foil and bake for twenty-five minutes. Uncover the apples then bake for another twenty to thirty minutes until the apples are soft and have risen.

Tip: Try substituting the apple with a pear.

GLUTEN-FREE COOKIE

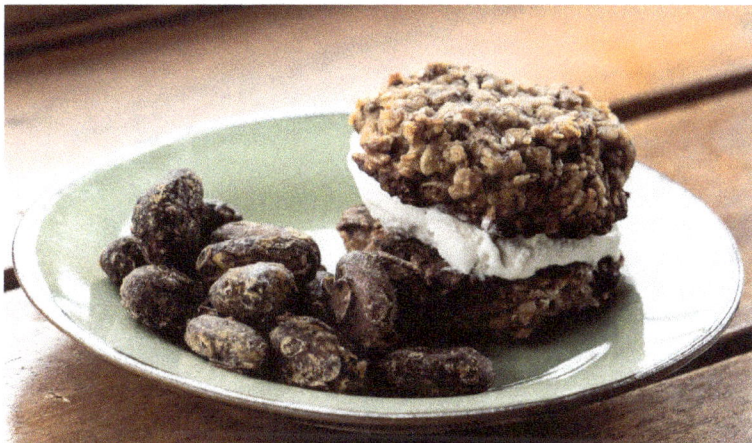

1 cup gluten-free, rolled oats. You can substitute quinoa flakes.
1 cup granola (make your own using the recipe on page 84)
2 large ripe bananas, mashed
¼ cup chocolate chips, seeds or nuts of your choice (optional)

1   Preheat the oven to 180 °C (350 °f). line a large cookie sheet with parchment paper and set aside.

2   Add all ingredients to a large mixing bowl and mix very well. If using chocolate chips, nuts, or seeds, stir them in with a spatula.

3   Form eight balls with the cookies. Place each ball on the cookie sheet and press each ball into a cookie shape. Bake for ten to twelve minutes, until slightly golden on the edges. Remove from the oven.

4   Allow cookies to cool for fifteen minutes before transferring to a wire rack to cool completely.

Tip: Cookies should be refrigerated and will keep for five days. They are freezer-friendly for up to two months. If you have an ice cream maker, you can try making ice cream sandwiches with vegan coconut milk. Or just serve with your favorite ice cream.

DARK CHOCOLATE BARK

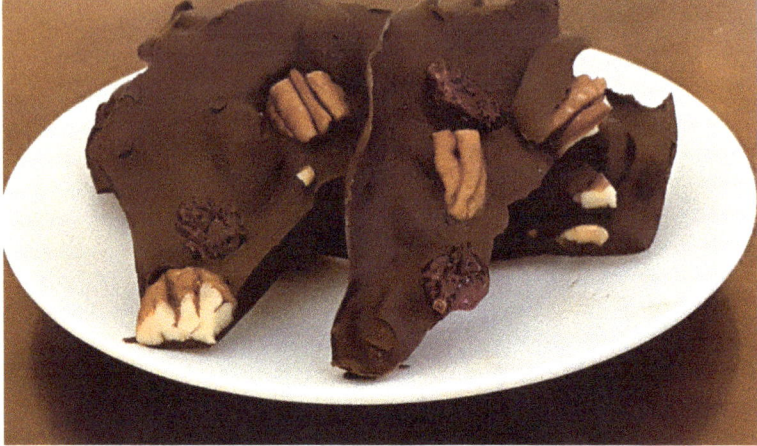

2 cups dark chocolate (60–70 percent cacao)
½ teaspoon coconut oil
½ cup roasted almonds or nut of your choice
½ tablespoon sea salt

1   Line a baking sheet with parchment paper. Using a sharp knife, finely chop the chocolate.
2   In a saucepan, on low, add chocolate and stir often, until the chocolate is completely melted and the mixture is smooth. Keep the heat on low the entire time. Be certain to remove the chocolate from the heat the moment it is melted or the texture will change.
3   Stir the nuts into the chocolate and spread onto the prepared baking sheet in a 1 cm (½ in) thick layer. Sprinkle with the sea salt. Place the chocolate bark in the fridge or freezer to cool, until hardened. Remove and break into pieces.

Tip: Substitute nuts with seeds and dried fruit of your choice.

FRUIT SALAD

VEGAN

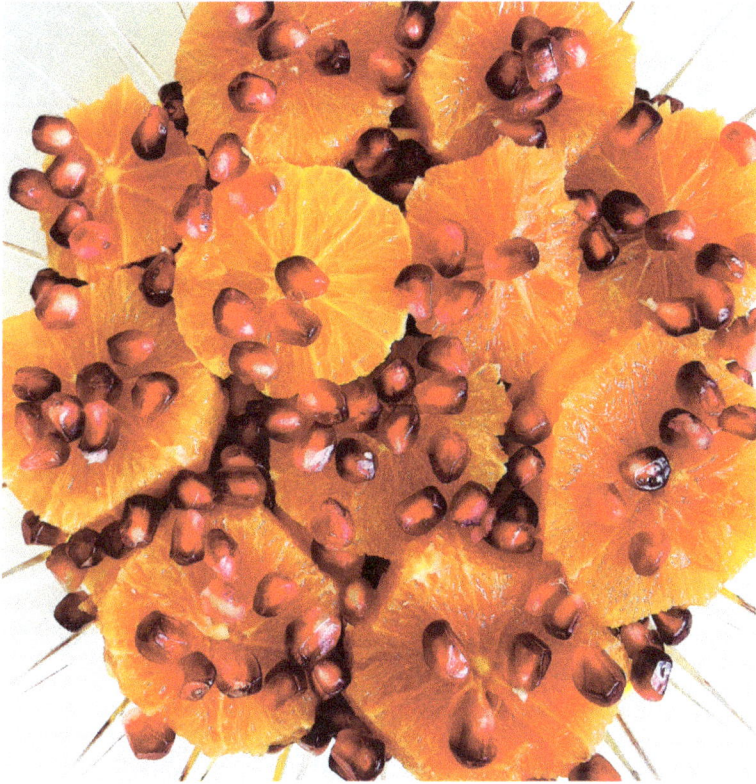

4 blood oranges
½ cup pomegranate seeds

Peel and slice oranges and sprinkle with pomegranate seeds.

Tip: I sometimes make my fruit salad with pineapple, mango and pomegranate seeds. I love the pop of the red seeds.

ENERGY BALLS

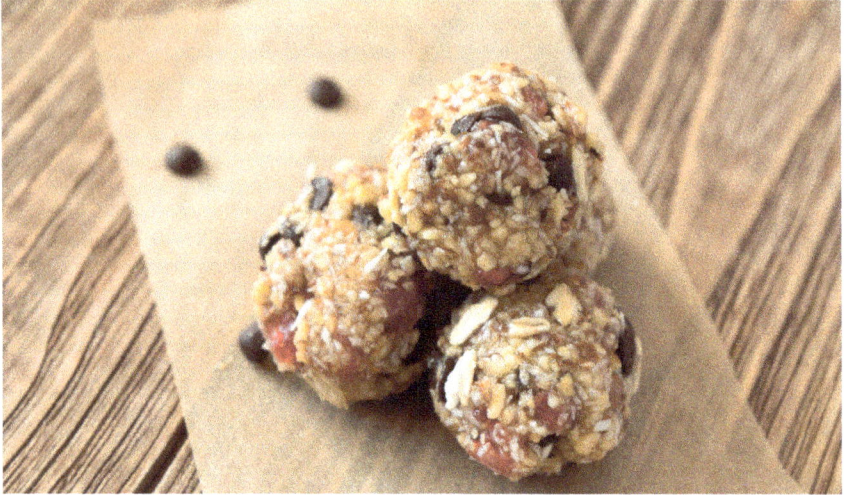

½ cup natural nut/seed butter

1 tablespoon honey

1¼ cups gluten-free oats

⅓ cup granola (make your own using the recipe on page 84)

½ cup dark chocolate chips

Combine the ingredients and roll into bite-size balls. Refrigerate until firm (about one hour).

Tip: Add nuts, seeds, or dried fruit of your choice instead of dark chocolate.

Here's to a Long, Healthy Life

My hope is that using this book will turn a possibility into a reality. It's here to give you a sense of empowerment as you make these small lifestyle changes and begin to reap the rewards, from eating a clean diet rich in whole foods, to making time for daily movement and learning to minimize stress in your life.

Appreciating and enjoying the food we eat is one way to experience happiness. In the rush of life, we often don't take the time to pause and enjoy the food Mother Nature provides for us. The way we nourish ourselves physically not only contributes to our own wellbeing but also impacts the web of life on this planet we share.

Food is medicine. It is what nourishes our bodies and increases longevity. Our overall health can be promoted by exercising regularly, reducing stress, and eating a primarily plant-based diet.

I encourage you to share your knowledge of a clean lifestyle and healthy foods through the recipes here to bring health into the life of your loved ones.

Acknowledgments

In my life there have been certain people who have been my mentors, friends, or sages whose presence has so deeply influenced my journey and inspired me to write this book.

I'd like to thank my cousin Chuck Hughes and my mother, Louise Hebert, for sharing tasty recipes.

Thank you to all the wonderful women who shared inspiring real-life stories, Lisa Burchartz, Virginia Harper, Sujatha Sundaram, MD, and the Grammar Factory team for helping this book come to life.

This book is dedicated to my children, John and Kate. Huge thank you for being part of this wonderful journey with me. They provide me the most profound experience, which is the most powerful healing medicine: unconditional love.

Bibliography

American Cancer Society. *Cancer Prevention & Early Detection Facts and Figures.* Atlanta: American Cancer Society, 2007.

Buettner, Dan. *The Blue Zones, Second Edition: 9 Lessons for Living Longer from the People Who've Lived the Longest.* Washington, D.C.: National Geographic, 2012.

Christakis, Nicholas A., and James H. Fowler. "The Spread of Obesity in a Large Social Network over 32 Years." *New England Journal of Medicine* 357, no. 4 (2007): 370–379. https://doi.org/10.1056/NEJMsa066082.

Environmental Working Group. "EWG's Skin Deep Cosmetic Database." https://www. ewg.org/skindeep/.

Environmental Working Group. "EWG's Shopper's Guide to Pesticides in Produce." https://www.ewg.org/foodnews/.

Harper, Virgina, and Tom Monte. *Controlling Crohn's Disease: The Natural Way.* Kensington Publishing Corporation, 2002.

Junger, Alejandro, and Amely Greven. *Clean: The Revolutionary Program to Restore the Body's Natural Ability to Heal Itself.* HarperOne, 2009.

Kushi, Michio, Stephen Blauer, and Wendy Esko. *The Macrobiotic Way: The Definitive Guide to Macrobiotic Living.* Avery, 2004.

Mayo Clinic. "Diabetes and Alzheimer's linked." Updated May 22, 2019. https:// www.mayoclinic.org/diseases-conditions/type-2-diabetes/in-depth/ diabetes-and-alzheimers/art-20046987.

The National Qigong Association. https:// www.nqa.org.

Schroeder, Elizabeth C., Warren D. Franke, Rick L. Sharp, Duck-chul Lee. "Comparative effectiveness of aerobic, resistance, and combined training on cardiovascular disease risk factors: A randomized controlled trial." *PLoS One* 14, no. 1 (2019). https://doi.org/10.1371/journal. pone.0210292.

Tolle, Eckhart. *The Power of Now: A Guide to Spiritual Enlightenment.* New World Library, 2004.

Tolle, Eckhart. *A New World: Awakening to Your Life's Purpose.* Penguin Books, 2016.

U.S. Food & Drug Administration. "Advice about Eating Fish: For Women Who Are or Might Become Pregnant, Breastfeeding Mothers, and Young Children." Updated August 31, 2020. https:// www.fda.gov/food/consumers/ advice-about-eating-fish

World Health Organization. "Water sanitation hygiene: Drinking-water quality guidelines." https://www. who.int/ water_sanitation_health/ water-quality/ guidelines/en/.

Yoga Journal. https://www.yogajournal. com.

About the Author

Lotus Ellis is the owner and founder of Lotus Fine Foods Inc and Lotus Fine Living Ltd. She has been in the health and wellness sector for two decades.

Her passion is to help people struggling with low energy and health setbacks make the connection between diet, life choices, and their health symptoms.

Spending six months living in Costa Rica completing RYT 200 yoga instructor training raised Lotus's understanding of the benefits of meditation and chakra balancing.

Lotus holds a Nutritional Certificate from Cornell University and has also studied both Ayurveda and macrobiotic principles. Her work brings together the best of old world therapies and modern nutrition to help heal the gut, lower inflammation, and boost immunity.

www.ingramcontent.com/pod-product-compliance
Lightning Source LLC
Chambersburg PA
CBHW052116030426
42335CB00025B/3011